...tric Imaging Cases

Pediatric Imaging Cases

Ellen Chung, MD
Chief, Radiologic Pathology
Walter Reed National Military Medical
Center at Bethesda
and
Pediatric Radiology Section Head
American Institute for Radiologic Pathology
and
Assistant Professor of Radiology and Pediatrics
Uniformed Services University
Bethesda, Maryland

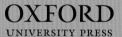

OXFORD
UNIVERSITY PRESS

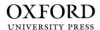

Oxford University Press is a department of the University of Oxford.
It furthers the University's objective of excellence in research, scholarship, and
education by publishing worldwide.

Oxford   New York
Auckland   Cape Town   Dar es Salaam   Hong Kong   Karachi
Kuala Lumpur   Madrid   Melbourne   Mexico City   Nairobi
New Delhi   Shanghai   Taipei   Toronto

With offices in
Argentina   Austria   Brazil   Chile   Czech Republic   France   Greece
Guatemala   Hungary   Italy   Japan   Poland   Portugal   Singapore
South Korea   Switzerland   Thailand   Turkey   Ukraine   Vietnam

Oxford is a registered trade mark of Oxford University Press in the UK
and certain other countries.

Published in the United States of America by
Oxford University Press
198 Madison Avenue, New York, NY 10016

Library of Congress Cataloging-in-Publication Data
    Chung, Ellen. Pediatric imaging cases / Ellen Chung.
      p. ; cm. — (Cases in radiology) (Cases in radiology)
    Includes bibliographical references and index.
    ISBN 978-0-19-975896-8 (pbk. : alk. paper)
    I. Title.   II. Series: Cases in radiology. [DNLM: 1. Diagnostic Imaging—methods—Case Reports.
    2. Diagnostic Imaging—methods—Examination Questions.   3. Child.   4. Infant.   5. Pediatrics—
    methods—Case Reports.   6. Pediatrics—methods—Examination Questions. WN 18.2]
    618.92′007575—dc23
    2012006843

9 8 7 6 5 4 3 2 1
Printed in China
on acid-free paper

To Kevin, Patricia, Diana, Shayna and the extended
Fellowplex for all your encouragement and
support and for making my life so rich

Preface

I have been collecting interesting cases since I was an intern, and my time at the Armed Forces Institute of Pathology allowed me to see a tremendous number of fascinating cases donated by the residents attending the rad-path course. This casebook allows me to share some of these with a wider audience. The hardest part of writing this book was selecting a group of cases that is relevant to most practices and that best represents the unique aspects of the subspecialty. I hope that this book proves helpful to those who occasionally care for children and sparks a greater interest in some readers to pursue further training in the fascinating and rewarding field of pediatric radiology.

Acknowledgments

Many stellar radiologists contributed to the cases in this book. I would like to acknowledge the following friends and colleagues for their contributions: Veronica Rooks, MD, COL, MC, US Army; Rajesh Krishnamurthy, MD; David Biko, MD, MAJ, US Air Force, MC; Jeanne Chow, MD; Jason Schroeder, MD, LCDR, US Navy; William R. Carter, MD, CDR, US Navy; Paul Clark, MD, MAJ, MC, US Army; Mark Murphey, MD; and Michael Callahan, MD. I would also like to recognize the many radiology residents who contributed cases to the archives of the Armed Forces Institute of Pathology.

The Publisher thanks the following for their time and advice:

Mark Anderson, University of Virginia
Sanjeev Bhalla, Mallinckrodt Institute of Radiology, Washington University
Michael Bruno, Penn State Hershey Medical Center
Melissa Rosado de Christenson, St. Luke's Hospital of Kansas City
Rihan Khan, University of Arizona
Angela Levy, Georgetown University
Alexander Mamourian, University of Pennsylvania
Stacy Smith, Brigham and Women's Hospital

Contents

Part 1   Cardiovascular System

History

▶ 5-month-old.

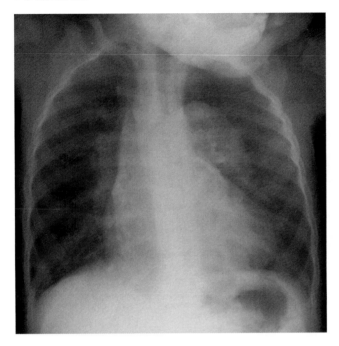

Case 1 Tetralogy of Fallot with Absent Pulmonary Valve

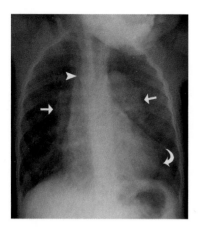

Findings

▸ PA chest radiograph shows a right aortic arch (arrowhead) causing a right-sided impression on the trachea. The cardiac silhouette is enlarged with an upturned apex (curved arrow). Bilateral massively enlarged central pulmonary arteries are seen (arrows) with decreased peripheral pulmonary vascularity.

Differential diagnosis

Other congenital cardiac anomalies are associated with right aortic arch, including truncus arteriosus, transposition of the great arteries, and tricuspid atresia.

Teaching points

▸ Tetralogy of Fallot (TOF) is the most common form of cyanotic congenital heart disease. The anomalies that make up TOF all result from anterior, superior, and leftward displacement of the conal septum causing right ventricular outflow obstruction, perimembranous ventricular septal defect (VSD), aorta overriding the VSD, and right ventricular hypertrophy. The pulmonary valve is often bicuspid or deficient.

▸ The degree of right ventricular outflow obstruction and the size of right-to-left shunts determine the clinical severity of the defect. With mild outflow obstruction and a large VSD, the patient may not appear clinically cyanotic ("pink tet"), although he may have episodes of cyanosis relieved by squatting to increase systemic resistance in order to increase pulmonary blood flow ("tet spells"). In the most severe form, the pulmonary outflow tract is atretic or even discontinuous (pseudo-truncus) and pulmonary blood flow is dependent on a patent ductus arteriosus and major aortopulmonary collateral arteries (MAPCAs). In absent pulmonary valve syndrome, there is massive dilation of the central pulmonary arteries in addition to the findings of TOF.

Next steps in management

TOF is now generally treated with a one-step total repair in infancy consisting of a transannular patch of the right ventricular outflow tract and closure of the VSD.

Further reading

1. Owens CM, Rees P, Elliot M, Shaw D. Plain chest radiographic images of the absent pulmonary valve syndrome. Br J Radiol. 1994 Mar;67(795):248–251.
2. Boechat MI, Ratib O, Williams PL, et al. Cardiac MR imaging and MR angiography for assessment of complex tetralogy of Fallot and pulmonary atresia. Radiographics. 2005 Nov–Dec;25(6):1535–1546.

History

▶ 9-year-old.

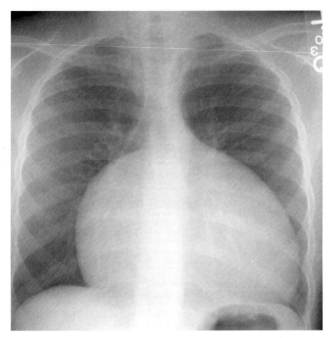

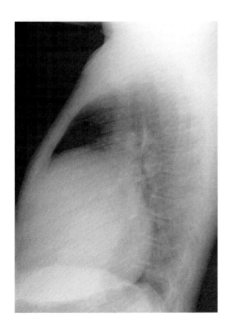

Case 2   Ebstein Anomaly

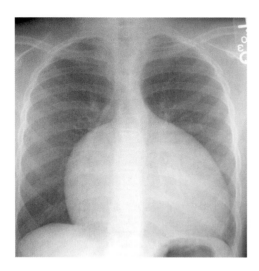 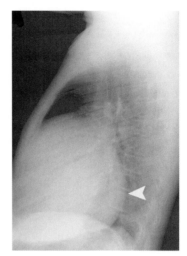

Findings

► PA chest radiograph (left) shows a markedly enlarged, globular or box-shaped heart and decreased pulmonary vascularity.
► The lateral view (right) shows the enlarged heart extending over the vertebral bodies (arrowhead).

Differential diagnosis

► Generally, decreased pulmonary blood flow is due to pulmonary outflow obstruction or tricuspid regurgitation. Simple tricuspid regurgitation and Uhl anomaly (absent right ventricular myocardium) should also be considered. Severe cardiac enlargement such as seen in this case is indicative of Ebstein anomaly.

Teaching points

► Ebstein anomaly is a rare cause of tricuspid regurgitation, accounting for less than 1% of cases of congenital heart defects. The septal and posterior leaflets of the tricuspid valve are malformed and displaced into the right ventricle. The anterior leaflet is normally positioned but may be redundant and sail-shaped. The result is division of the right ventricle into two chambers—the "atrialized" upper portion and the lower outflow portion. The valvular deformity causes severe tricuspid regurgitation and volume overload results in massive enlargement of the right heart, which in turn causes worsening of the tricuspid regurgitation.
► All patients also have an atrial septal defect or patent foramen ovale, and volume overload on the right side leads to right-to-left shunting across the atrial septum and resultant decrease in pulmonary blood flow.

Next steps in management

► Diagnosis is made on the basis of echocardiography. MR imaging shows the valvular malformation and can be used to evaluate RV function and to quantify the right-to-left shunt and degree of tricuspid regurgitation. Most patients present during the first month of life and the mortality is high. Initial supportive therapy consists of prostaglandin-E2 to maintain patency of the ductus arteriosus and extracorporeal membrane oxygenation as necessary while awaiting the normal resolution of perinatal high pulmonary vascular resistance.

Further reading

1. Ferguson EC, Krishnamurthy R, Oldham SA. Classic imaging signs of congenital cardiovascular abnormalities. Radiographics. 2007 Sep–Oct;27(5):1323–1334.
2. Waldman JD, Wenly JA. Cyanotic congenital heart disease with decreased pulmonary blood flow in children. Pediatr Clin North Am. 1999 Apr;46(2):385–404.

History

► Cyanotic newborn. Second image is post-operative.

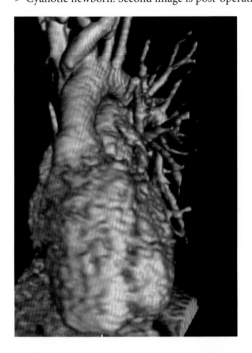

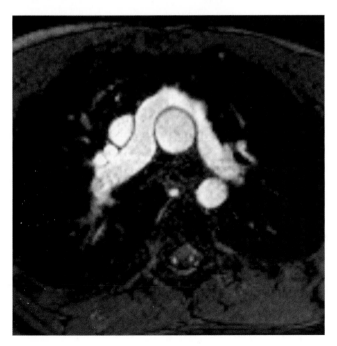

Case 3 Dextro-Transposition of the Great Arteries (D-TGA)

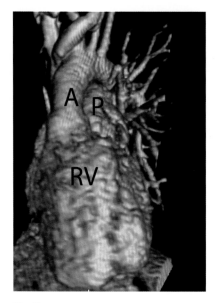
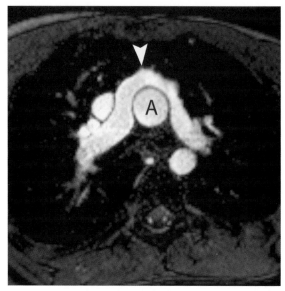

Findings

▶ Volume-rendered enhanced MR image viewed from anterior (left) shows the aorta (A) arising from the anterior right ventricle (RV) and to the right of the pulmonary artery (P).

▶ Postoperative image shows the switched pulmonary artery (arrowhead) draped over the ascending aorta (A).

Differential diagnosis

Other conotruncal anomalies should be considered.

Teaching points

▶ Using the segmental approach, the first step is determination of visceroatrial situs, or the position of the atria relative to other organs (see Case 8, Asplenia).

▶ Next, the orientation of the ventricular loop is determined. Normally, the cardiac tube folds to the right (D-loop) so that the right ventricle (RV) is to the right of the left ventricle (LV). The morphologic RV has coarse trabeculae and an apical moderator band. The LV is smooth.

▶ Third, the position of the origins of the great arteries is determined. Normally, the aorta originates posterior and to the right of the pulmonary artery (PA). In D-transposition, the aorta originates anterior and to the right of the PA. In L-transposition, the aorta is anterior and to the left of the PA.

▶ Next, the relationships between the atria and ventricles and between the ventricles and the great arteries are determined. D-TGA is ventriculo-arterial discordance. Deoxygenated blood is pumped to the systemic circulation, while oxygenated blood is returned to the lungs. Survival depends on mixing of blood through a shunt. In L-TGA, there is also ventriculo-atrial discordance with ventricular inversion (L-loop), so that the morphologic RV is on the left. Blood flow is appropriate, but the RV functions as the systemic ventricle.

Next steps in management

The preferred treatment is the Jatene arterial switch.

Further reading

1. Lapierre C, Déry J, Guérin R, et al. Segmental approach to imaging of congenital heart disease. Radiographics. 2010 Mar; 30(2):397–411.
2. Dorfman AL, Geva T. Magnetic resonance imaging evaluation of congenital heart disease: conotruncal anomalies. J Cardiovasc Magn Reson. 2006;8(4):645–659.

History

▶ 4-year-old with abnormal chest radiograph.

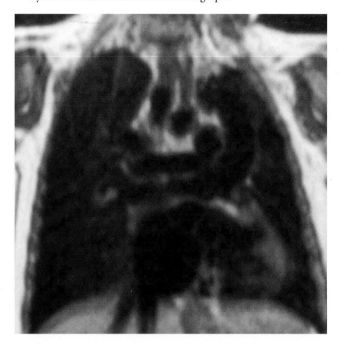

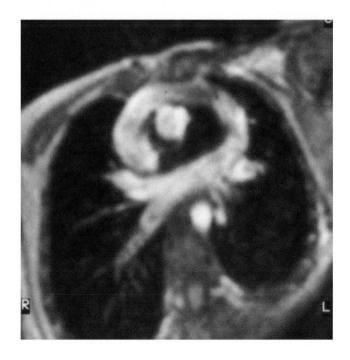

Case 4 Total Anomalous Pulmonary Venous Return (TAPVR)

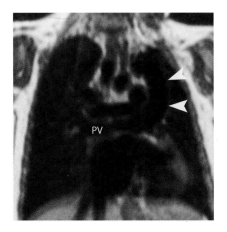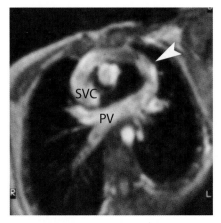

Findings

▶ Coronal T1-weighted image (left) reveals a large persistent vertical vein (arrowheads) between the right pulmonary vein (PV) and the left innominate vein.

▶ Oblique axial image from a gadolinium-enhanced MRA shows the anomalous vein (arrowhead) draining the PV into the left innominate vein to the superior vena cava (SVC).

Differential diagnosis

For nonobstructed TAPVR, the plain radiograph shows cardiac enlargement and increased pulmonary blood flow since the anomalous pulmonary venous drainage constitutes a left-to-right shunt. The differential diagnosis includes acyanotic left-to-right shunts. For obstructed TAPVR, the plain radiographs shows pulmonary edema, and the differential diagnosis includes left heart obstructing lesions.

Teaching points

▶ In total anomalous pulmonary venous return or connection, all pulmonary veins drain via anomalous vein(s) to the systemic venous system. An obligatory shunt at the atrial level allows mixing of oxygenated and deoxygenated blood.

▶ Four types are described based on the location of the systemic-anomalous venous connection: supracardiac, cardiac, infracardiac, and mixed. Clinically, patients are categorized as having either nonobstructed or obstructed pulmonary venous flow. Obstructed patients present in the neonatal period.

▶ In the supracardiac type, the pulmonary veins drain into the persistent vertical vein, which forms a rounded left superior mediastinal border. Without obstruction to pulmonary venous drainage, the superior vena cava is enlarged from blood shunted from the left, and forms a rounded right mediastinal border. The cardiomediastinal silhouette resembles a snowman.

▶ The infracardiac type frequently drains below the diaphragm and is almost always obstructed. The pulmonary vein passes through the esophageal hiatus, most commonly draining into the portal venous system, and the obstruction is at the level of the hepatic sinusoids.

Next steps in management

MRI/MRA is helpful for cardiac-level lesions and in the evaluation of right ventricular function.

Further reading

1. Ferguson EC, Krishnamurthy R, Oldham SA. Classic imaging signs of congenital cardiovascular abnormalities. Radiographics. 2007 Sep–Oct;27(5):1323–1334.
2. Kellenberger CJ, Yoo SJ, Büchel ER. Cardiovascular MR imaging in neonates and infants with congenital heart disease. Radiographics. 2007:27:5–18.

History

▶ 5-day-old with murmur.

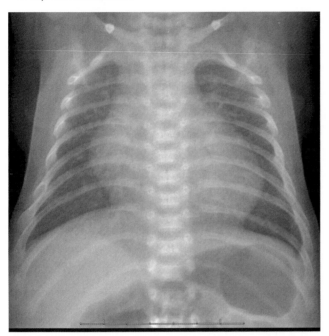

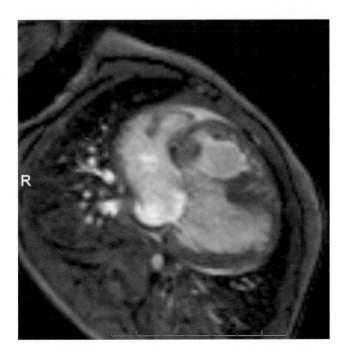

Case 5 Common Atrioventricular Canal (CAVC)

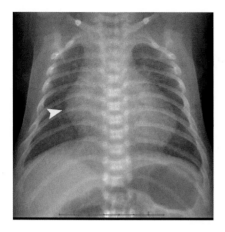 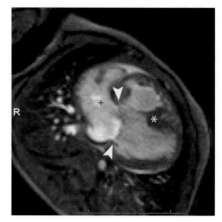

Findings

- ▶ PA chest radiograph (left) shows cardiomegaly with prominent right atrium (arrowhead).
- ▶ Four-chamber enhanced MR image (right) shows only the lower portion of the ventricular septum (*), communication of the atria (+), and common AV valve spanning the right and left heart (arrowheads).

Differential diagnosis

Acyanotic left-to-right shunts include other intracardiac shunts (see below) and extracardiac shunts (e.g., vein of Galen malformation and hepatic hemangioendothelioma).

Teaching points

- ▶ Ventricular septal defect (VSD) is the most common congenital heart defect excluding bicuspid aortic valve. Patients present in the neonatal period when the physiologic decrease in pulmonary vascular resistance leads to an increase in left-to-right shunting.
- ▶ Atrial septal defect (ASD) is also common and most likely to be diagnosed in an older child. The ostium secundum type is most common.
- ▶ CAVC, or atrioventricular septal defect, represents abnormal development of the endocardial cushion and is strongly associated with trisomy 21. A partial defect consists of an ostium primum ASD with clefts in the tricuspid and mitral valves. The complete defect includes the ASD and an inlet or canal-type VSD with a common, five-leaflet AV valve.
- ▶ Patent ductus arteriosus is more common in premature infants. Normally, the ductus closes functionally within the first 48 hours of life. Hypoxemia, as seen in premature infants with surfactant deficiency, inhibits closure.
- ▶ Chest radiographs show an enlarged heart and shunt vascularity, in which pulmonary arteries and veins are enlarged, but distinct. The right heart and left atrium are enlarged in CAVC and VSD, but the left atrium is not enlarged in ASD because it immediately decompresses into the right atrium.

Next steps in management

MRI is useful for quantifying the shunt and in follow-up. ASDs can be treated with percutaneous transcatheter placement of closure devices. Small VSDs close spontaneously. AV canal defects are closed surgically.

Further reading

1. Krishnamurthy R. Pediatric cardiac MRI: anatomy and function. Pediatr Radiol. 2008;38:S192–S199.
2. Wang ZJ, Reddy GP, Gotway MB, et al. Cardiovascular shunts: MR imaging evaluation. Radiographics 2003;23:Spec no. S181–S194.

History

▶ 5-year-old with hypertension.

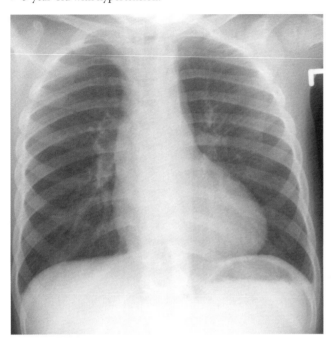

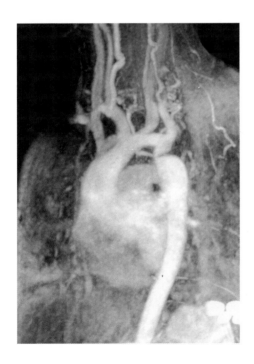

Case 6 Coarctation of the Aorta with Bicuspid Aortic Valve

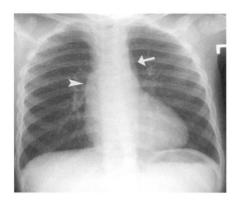 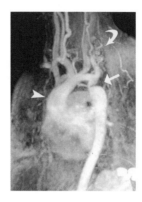

Findings

- PA chest radiograph shows a dilated, border-forming ascending aorta (arrowhead) due to turbulent flow through the stenotic aortic valve, and a subtle notch in the aortic knob (arrow).
- MIP image from gadolinium-enhanced MRA shows the dilated ascending aorta (arrowhead), the focal coarctation (arrow), and collateral vessels (curved arrow).

Differential diagnosis

Pseudo-coarctation describes an elongated aorta with a kink at the ligamentum arteriosum but without significant narrowing of the lumen. Collateral circulation is absent in pseudo-coarctation.

Teaching points

- Coarctation of the aorta is generally divided into two types:
  - Discrete or focal—a shelf-like narrowing that usually affects the isthmus just distal to the origin of the left subclavian artery
  - Diffuse—hypoplasia of a long segment (usually the transverse arch)
- The diffuse form is frequently associated with other anomalies and more commonly presents in infancy. Associations include bicuspid aortic valve, mitral valve anomalies, hypoplastic left heart syndrome (HLHS), and Turner syndrome.
- Critical coarctation presents at the end of the first week of life with acute decompensation accompanying closure of the ductus arteriosus, which further increases left ventricular afterload.
- The focal form is usually discovered incidentally on physical exam or chest radiography.
- Plain radiographic findings consist of the three-shaped aortic knob due to pre- and post-stenotic dilation. Rib notching due to enlarged intercostal collaterals is not seen prior to age 8 years.
- MRA with velocity-encoded cine phase contrast imaging can quantify the severity of the stenosis. The peak velocity in the descending aorta is determined and used to calculate the gradient across the stenosis.

Next steps in management

MRA is useful in preoperative planning and postoperative follow-up. Focal lesions are amenable to balloon dilation, while long stenoses are best treated surgically.

Further reading

1. Ferguson EC, Krishnamurthy R, Oldham SA. Classic imaging signs of congenital cardiovascular abnormalities. Radiographics. 2007 Sep–Oct;27(5):1323–1334.
2. Didier D, Saint-Martin C, Lapierre C, et al. Coarctation of the aorta: pre- and postoperative evaluation with echocardiography and surgery. Int J Cardiovasc Imaging 2006;22:457–475.

History

▶ 2-day-old with heart failure.

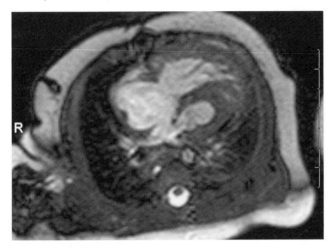

Case 7 Hypoplastic Left Heart Syndrome (HLHS)

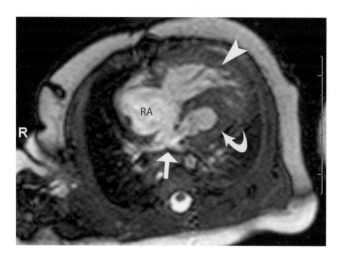

Findings

▸ Preoperative four-chamber view (left) shows a small left ventricle (curved arrow), normal right ventricle (arrowhead), small left atrium (arrow), and normal right atrium (RA).

Differential diagnosis

Congestive heart failure (CHF) in the infant may be caused by any left heart obstructing lesion, including (from distal to proximal) aortic coarctation, congenital aortic stenosis, HLHS, mitral stenosis, cor triatriatum, congenital pulmonary vein stenosis, and obstructive total anomalous pulmonary venous return.

Teaching points

▸ HLHS consists of hypoplasia of the left ventricle (LV) with inflow and outflow obstruction and represents the most common cause of CHF in the first week of life. In addition to LV hypoplasia, the ascending aorta is hypoplastic, the aortic and mitral valves are stenotic or atretic, and there is an obligatory intra-atrial left-to-right shunt. Most also have coarctation of the aorta. Systemic blood flow is ductus dependent.

▸ Patients present in the first week of life. Postpartum physiologic changes precipitate rapid clinical decline. The normal decrease in pulmonary arterial resistance causes more left-to-right shunting and decreased systemic perfusion. Normal closure of the ductus further reduces systemic blood flow.

Next steps in management

MRI/MRA is helpful in surgical planning and follow-up for all stages of palliative repair. Stage I (Norwood procedure) consists of separation of the main pulmonary artery from the right and left branches, anastomosis of the main pulmonary artery (PA) to the aorta so that the right ventricle becomes the systemic as well as the pulmonary ventricle, reconstruction of the hypoplastic ascending aorta, atrial septectomy to facilitate flow of oxygenated and deoxygenated blood to the solitary functioning ventricle, and creation of a modified Blalock-Taussig shunt to supply the pulmonary arteries. In the stage II procedure, the superior vena cava is anastomosed to the PA. In the stage III correction (Fontan procedure), a shunt is created from the inferior vena cava to the PA so that all systemic venous flow reaches the PA passively.

Further reading

1. Krishnamurthy R. Pediatric cardiac MRI: anatomy and function. Pediatr Radiol. 2008;38:S192–S199.
2. Bardo DM, Frankel DG, Applegate KE, et al. Hypoplastic left heart syndrome. Radiographics. 2001;221:705–717.

History

▶ Newborn with respiratory distress.

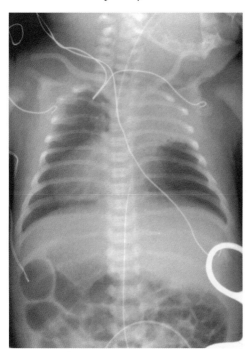

Case 8   Asplenia

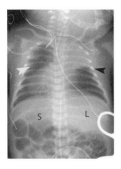

Findings

▶ AP radiograph demonstrates an endotracheal tube. The heart and cardiac apex are on the right. The stomach (S) is on the right and the liver (L) is on the left. The thymus is involuted and no right-sided aortic arch is seen. Left upper lobe atelectasis borders a left minor fissure (black arrowhead). A right minor fissure is also seen (white arrowhead).

Differential diagnosis

Asplenia is part of a highly variable spectrum of abnormalities known as heterotaxy syndrome.

Teaching points

▶ The systemic or morphologic right atrium is the one that receives blood return from the vena cavae and has a wide-based atrial appendage. The pulmonary or morphologic left atrium receives blood return from the lungs and has a finger-like atrial appendage. The right bronchus is short and eparterial (above the right pulmonary artery), while the left is longer and hyparterial.

▶ Situs solitus is the normal arrangement of chest and abdominal organs. Situs inversus totalis is the complete mirror image of situs solitus. The incidence of congenital heart disease (CHD) with situs inversus totalis is slightly higher than normal (3–5%).

▶ All other arrangements are known as *situs ambiguous* or *heterotaxy syndrome*. Some of these patients fall into the specific subsets known as *asplenia* and *polysplenia*.

▶ Asplenia or bilateral right-sidedness consists of bilateral trilobed lungs and eparterial bronchi, bilateral systemic atria, absent spleen, midline liver, and variable stomach. The incidence of CHD is nearly 100% (usually transposition).

▶ Polysplenia or bilateral left-sidedness consists of bilateral bilobed lungs and hyparterial bronchi, bilateral pulmonary atria, many small spleens, midline or left liver, variable stomach, and usually interruption of the inferior vena cava with azygos continuation. The incidence of CHD is much lower in polysplenia.

Next steps in management

Imaging of suspected situs abnormality should include the following: echocardiography; ultrasound of the abdomen; and upper GI series to evaluate for malrotation.

Further reading

1. Applegate KE, Goske MJ, Pierce G, Murphy D. Situs revisited: imaging of the heterotaxy syndrome. Radiographics. 1999 Jul–Aug;19(4):837–852.
2. Winer-Muram HT, Tonkin IL. The spectrum of heterotaxic syndromes. Radiol Clin North Am. 1989;27: 1147–1170.

History

▶ 3-month-old boy with biphasic stridor.

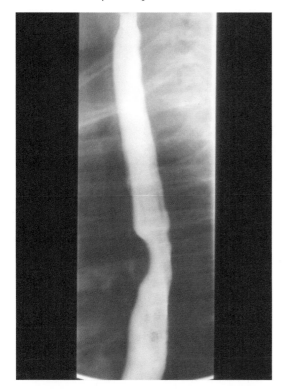

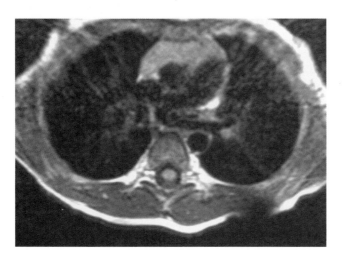

Case 9   Pulmonary Sling

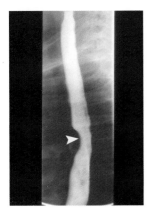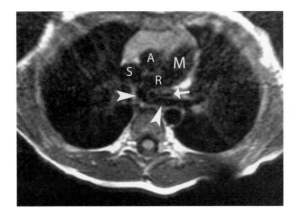

Findings

▶ Lateral image from an esophagram (left) shows an anterior impression on the mid-esophagus (arrowhead).

▶ Axial black-blood T1-weighted image shows the main pulmonary artery (M) with only a right branch (R). The left pulmonary artery originates from the right and crosses behind the trachea (arrow) to get to the left side (arrowheads). (S = superior vena cava, A = aorta)

Differential diagnosis

The aortic vascular rings cause posterior impressions on the esophagus at the level of the aortic arch.

Teaching points

▶ In pulmonary sling, or anomalous pulmonary artery, the left pulmonary artery originates from the right rather than directly from the main pulmonary artery.

▶ The anomalous pulmonary artery crosses between the trachea and esophagus just above the carina to get to the left side. This causes an anterior impression on the esophagus and a posterior impression on the trachea and forms a sling around the trachea.

▶ The ductus arteriosus extends from the origin of the right pulmonary artery to the post-subclavian aorta, forming a complete ring around the trachea only.

▶ Patients commonly present with respiratory difficulties due to associated airway abnormalities.

- The anomalous vessel compresses the bronchus intermedius, causing air trapping or atelectasis in the right middle and lower lobes.
- Tracheomalacia—collapse of the trachea in exhalation
- Complete tracheal rings—causes long segment severe tracheal stenosis and significant morbidity and mortality
- T-shaped trachea—low obtuse carina of no clinical import

▶ Associated with pulmonary lobation abnormalities, tracheal bronchus, and congenital heart disease

Next steps in management

MRA or CTA is performed preoperatively.

Further reading

1. Newman B, Cho Y. Left pulmonary artery sling—anatomy and imaging. Semin Ultrasound CT MR. 2010;31:158–170.
2. Lee KY, Yoon CS, Choe KO, et al. Use of imaging for assessing anatomical relationships of tracheobronchial anomalies associated with left pulmonary artery sling. Pediatr Radiol. 2001;31:269–278.

History

► 4-year-old boy with dysphagia.

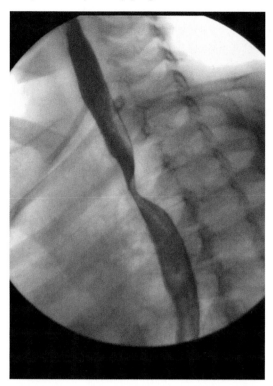

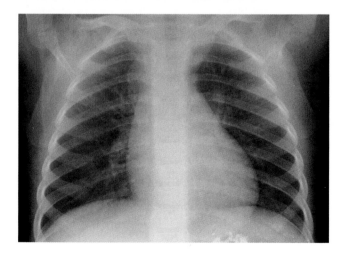

Case 10   Right Aortic Arch with Aberrant Left Subclavian Artery

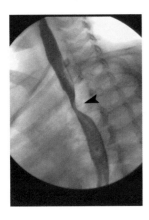 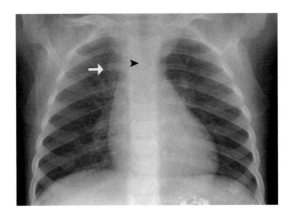

Findings

▶ Lateral view from an esophagram demonstrates a posterior impression on the esophagus (arrowhead).

▶ AP chest radiograph (right) reveals a right aortic arch (arrow) causing a right-sided impression on the trachea (arrowhead).

Differential diagnosis

The differential diagnosis for the posterior impression on the esophagus includes left arch with aberrant right subclavian artery (a normal variant) and double aortic arch.

Teaching points

▶ The two complete aortic rings are right arch with aberrant left subclavian artery (LSCA) and double aortic arch. These account for the majority of symptomatic vascular rings and both have a right aortic arch.

▶ The evaluation of an infant with stridor/wheeze or dysphagia begins with chest radiographs. The finding of a normal left arch virtually excludes a complete aortic ring.

▶ The aortic arch may be obscured by the thymus on the chest radiograph in an infant. The best way to determine the side of the aortic arch is by observing the mass effect (impression) of the arch on the trachea.

▶ The next step is an esophagram. A posterior impression on the esophagus at the level of the arch indicates the presence of an aberrant subclavian artery or two arches joining posteriorly.

▶ In right arch with aberrant LSCA, there are four, rather than three, branches of the aortic arch. The last branch is the LSCA, which originates on the right side and crosses posterior to the esophagus to get to the left side, causing the posterior impression on the esophagus.

▶ In double aortic arch there is a posterior impression and bilateral lateral (three impressions) on the esophagus and there are bilateral lateral impressions on the trachea (the right is usually larger).

Next steps in management

MRA or CTA for preoperative planning if symptomatic.

Further reading

1. Kellenberger CJ. Aortic arch malformations. Pediatr Radiol. Jun;40(6):876–884.
2. Russo V, Renzulli M, La Palombara C, Fattori R. Congenital disease of the thoracic aorta. Role of MRI and MRA. Eur Radiol. 2006 Mar;16(3):676–684.

History

▶ 10-year-old girl with dyspnea on exertion.

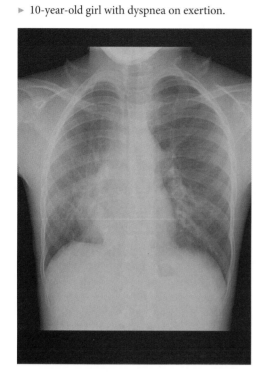

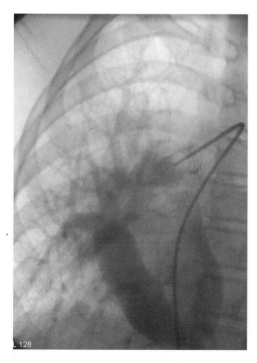

Case 11 Scimitar Syndrome

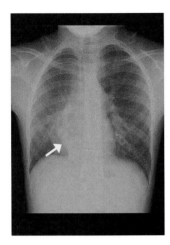 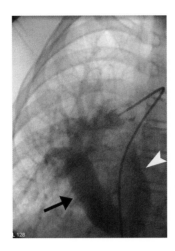

Findings

▶ PA chest radiograph (left) reveals a slightly small right lung with shift of the heart and mediastinum to the right. Additionally, a retrocardiac tubular density (arrow) is noted coursing toward the right hemidiaphragm.

▶ AP image obtained in the venous phase of a pulmonary angiogram shows that the tubular structure is a large pulmonary vein (arrow) that drains via the inferior vena cava to the right atrium (arrowhead).

Differential diagnosis

The findings are diagnostic but associated anomalies should be considered, particularly in children.

Teaching points

▶ Scimitar syndrome, also known by the broader term "pulmonary venolobar syndrome," is a form of partial anomalous pulmonary venous return. The right lower lobe, or a portion of the right lower lobe, is drained by a large vein (called *scimitar* vein because of its resemblance to a Turkish sword) that courses toward the diaphragm. Instead of draining into the left atrium as a normal pulmonary vein would, the scimitar vein drains into the right atrium, and thus represents a left-to-right shunt.

▶ The term "pulmonary venolobar syndrome" encompasses the additional component of hypogenetic right lung. Consequent radiologic findings include dextroposition of the heart and so-called alveolar tissue seen anterior to the right lobe on the lateral view.

▶ Additional associated abnormalities may include pulmonary sequestration, absence of the pulmonary artery with systemic arterialization of the lung, absence of the inferior vena cava, accessory diaphragm, horseshoe lung, and congenital cardiac anomalies.

▶ CT angiography is useful in the preoperative evaluation of symptomatic children with complex anomalies.

Next steps in management

Most patients require no therapy, but symptomatic children with complex anomalies may require endovascular or surgical intervention.

Further reading

1. Konen E, Raviv-Zilka L, Cohen RA, et al. Congenital pulmonary venolobar syndrome: spectrum of helical CT findings with emphasis on computerized reformatting. Radiographics. 2003 Sep–Oct;23(5):1175–1184.
2. Woodring JH, Howard TA, Kanga JF. Congenital pulmonary venolobar syndrome revisited. Radiographics 1994; 14:349–369.

Part 2   Gastrointestinal System

History

► 2-month-old with persistent neonatal jaundice.

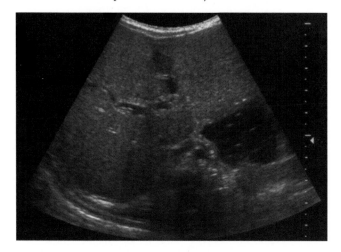

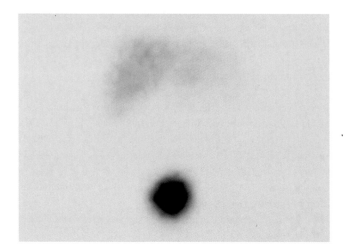

Case 12 Biliary Atresia

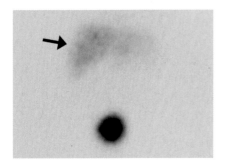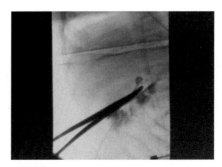

Findings

▶ The ultrasound (previous page) showed no extrahepatic bile ducts or gallbladder. Sixty-minute image from hepatobiliary scintigraphy (left) shows hepatic (arrow) and bladder activity, but no bowel activity.

▶ Intraoperative cholangiogram (right) shows no intrahepatic biliary ducts.

Differential diagnosis

The main differential diagnostic consideration for a jaundiced infant is neonatal hepatitis. Hepatobiliary scintigraphy in neonatal hepatitis may also demonstrate absence of excretion into the bowel due to hepatocellular dysfunction. Premedication with phenobarbital for 5 days allows bowel excretion in patients with neonatal hepatitis, preventing a false-positive result. Another differential consideration is choledochal cyst, although 8% to 11% of cases of biliary atresia are associated with portal cysts.

Teaching points

▶ Ultrasound findings of biliary atresia include absence of a normal gallbladder in an infant who has been fasted for at least 4 hours. A small gallbladder may be seen with biliary atresia. The triangular cord sign is a triangular echogenic focus more than 4 mm in thickness at the anterior wall of the right portal vein above the portal bifurcation, representing a fibrotic extrahepatic biliary duct. This sign is very specific and is considered diagnostic in conjunction with an abnormal (short or absent) gallbladder.

▶ In biliary atresia, hepatobiliary scintigraphy using Tc99m-DISIDA demonstrates absence of enteric excretion of radiopharmaceutical by 1 hour and on 24-hour delayed imaging.

▶ Magnetic resonance cholangiopancreatography (MRCP) may demonstrate a patent extrahepatic bilary duct, a finding that excludes the diagnosis of biliary atresia.

▶ In equivocal cases, intraoperative cholangiography may be necessary to confirm the diagnosis.

Next steps in management

The initial treatment of choice is the Kasai hepatic portoenterostomy, which is most likely to achieve successful biliary drainage if performed prior to age 3 to 4 months.

Further reading

1. Rozel C, Garel L, Rypens R, et al. Imaging of liver disorders in children. Pediatr Radiol. 2010 Sep; 24 epub.
2. Lee MS, Kim MJ, Lee, MJ, et al. Biliary atresia: color Doppler US findings in neonates and infants. Radiology 2009 July;252(1):282–289.

History

▶ 2-year-old girl with jaundice.

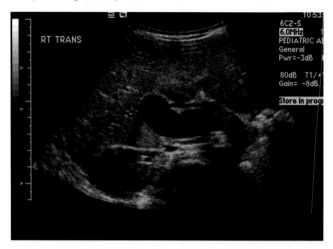

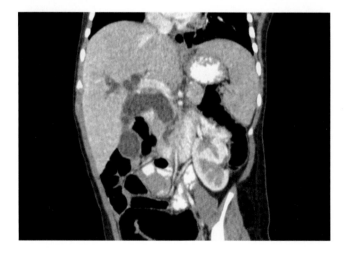

Case 13 Choledochal Cyst

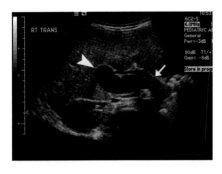 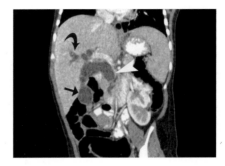

Findings

▶ Transverse ultrasound image (left) reveals a tubular cyst in the porta hepatis (arrowhead), extending to the pancreas (arrow).

▶ CT coronal reconstruction (right) shows the tubular cyst (arrowhead), dilated intrahepatic ducts (curved arrow), and a distinct gallbladder (arrow).

Differential diagnosis

Other cystic lesions in the pediatric abdomen include enteric duplication cyst, mesenteric cyst, lymphatic malformation, ureteropelvic junction obstruction, multicystic dysplastic kidney, and mature cystic teratoma. The choledochal cyst may be distinguished by its location in the porta hepatis, communication with bile ducts, absence of gut signature in the wall, and tubular configuration.

Teaching points

▶ Choledochal cysts are four times more common in females. They are often congenital, but in older children and adults, choledochal cysts may be acquired due to an abnormally long common hepatic-pancreatic duct that allows reflux of pancreatic enzymes into the common bile duct.

▶ Coexisting biliary atresia should be considered in young infants with persistent neonatal jaundice and a cyst in the porta hepatis. Complications include stone formation, cholangitis, biliary cirrhosis, and cholangiocarcinoma.

▶ Type 1 is dilation of the extrahepatic duct and is the most common (80–90%). Type 2 is a diverticulum of the bile duct. Type 3 is a choledochocele herniating into the duodenal wall. Type 4 is multiple intrahepatic and/or extrahepatic cysts. Type 5 is Caroli disease (intrahepatic duct dilation without obstruction).

▶ On ultrasound, a cyst is seen in the porta hepatis separate from the gallbladder and communicating with bile ducts. Choledocholithiasis or echogenic debris may be noted. On magnetic resonance cholangiopancreatography (MRCP), the cyst and its relationship to bile ducts are well demonstrated. Hepatobiliary scintigraphy generally demonstrates accumulation of radiopharmaceutical in the cyst and drainage into the bowel.

Next steps in management

Treatment is surgical excision of the entire cyst with reconstruction of biliary-enteric drainage.

Further reading

1. Rozel C, Garel L, Rypens R, et al. Imaging of liver disorders in children. Pediatr Radiol. 2011 Feb; 42(2):208–220.
2. Chavhan GB, Babyn PS, Manson D, Vidarsson L. Pediatric MR cholangiopancreatography: principles, technique, and clinical applications. Radiographics 2008 Nov–Dec;28(7):1951–1962.

History

▶ Newborn with mass.

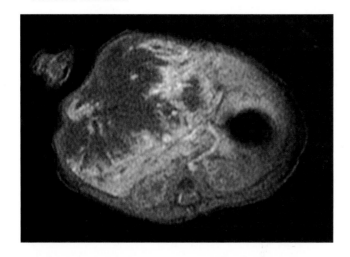

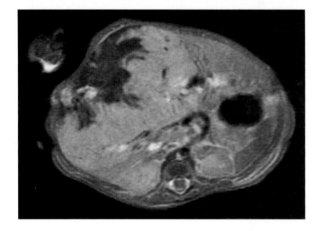

Case 14 Infantile Hepatic Hemangioendothelioma

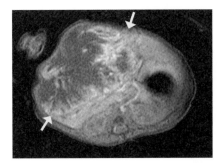 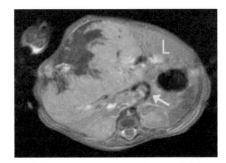

Findings

▶ Early-phase enhanced axial T1-weighted image (left) shows a mass with intense, irregular peripheral enhancement (arrows).

▶ Delayed-phase axial T1-weighted image shows centripetal fill-in of enhancement and the large flow void of the celiac axis (arrow). L = adjacent liver.

Differential diagnosis

Other congenital hepatic tumors should be considered. Infantile hemangioendothelioma (IHE) can be distinguished from hepatoblastoma by its characteristic dynamic enhancement pattern and by the absence of elevated levels of serum AFP. IHE and metastatic neuroblastoma can both appear as multiple masses, but metastases enhance less than adjacent liver.

Teaching points

▶ IHE is the most common benign hepatic tumor of infancy. Most are diagnosed in the first few months of life. A vascular mass presenting after age 1 year is concerning for malignancy.

▶ Clinical complications may include high-output cardiac failure from shunting of blood flow to the tumor and the Kasabach-Merritt syndrome of tumoral platelet sequestration.

▶ Hemangiomas of the skin and other sites are present in up to 68% of patients.

▶ IHE is a high-flow vascular lesion, and evidence of high flow, such as enlarged vessels and decrease in the caliber of the aorta below the origin of the celiac axis, is frequently apparent.

▶ IHE may appear as a large solitary mass often with central hemorrhage, necrosis, or fibrosis, or as multiple smaller, uniform masses.

▶ Lesions are usually hypoechoic on ultrasound. Dynamic contrast-enhanced imaging reveals peripheral nodular or corrugated enhancement with progressive centripetal fill-in, which is incomplete due to central hemorrhage or fibrotic scar.

Next steps in management

Dynamic contrast-enhanced CT or MR is indicated to confirm the diagnosis. The symptomatic patient is treated medically, and all patients are followed closely with ultrasound to confirm resolution. Patients with arteriovenous shunting and life-threatening complications may require embolotherapy.

Further reading

1. Chung EM, Cube R, Lewis RB, et al. Pediatric liver masses: radiologic-pathologic correlation. Radiographics 2010;30:801–826.
2. Kassarjian A, Zurakowski D, Dubois J, et al. Infantile hepatic hemangiomas: clinical and imaging findings and their correlation with therapy. AJR Am J Roentgenol 2004;182(3):785–795.

History

▶ 10-month-old girl with worsening emesis and epigastric mass.

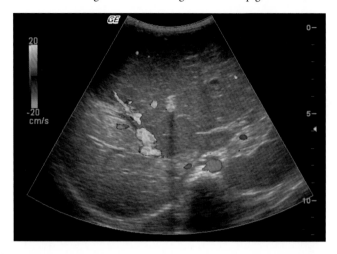

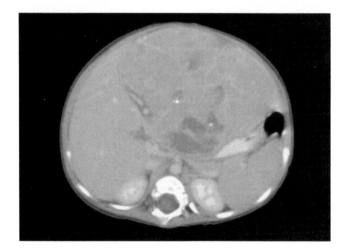

Case 15   Hepatoblastoma

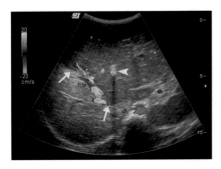 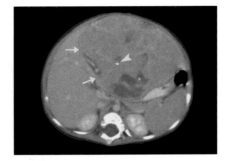

Findings

▶ A transverse color Doppler sonogram reveals a well-defined hypovascular, hypoechoic mass within the liver (arrows) with a shadowing echogenic calcification (arrowhead).

▶ Axial contrast-enhanced T1-weighted MR image shows a heterogeneous mass (arrows) with small calcifications (arrowhead).

Differential diagnosis

Other liver masses that occur in this age group include infantile hemangioendothelioma, mesenchymal hamartoma, and metastases (usually from neuroblastoma). Infantile hemangioendothelioma is a markedly hypervascular mass. Dynamic contrast-enhanced imaging studies demonstrate characteristic peripheral, nodular enhancement with progressive centripetal fill-in. Mesenchymal hamartoma is typically predominantly cystic while hepatoblastoma is mostly solid. Metastases are generally multiple rather than solitary masses and the primary is usually visible in the retroperitoneum, pelvis, or posterior mediastinum.

Teaching points

▶ Hepatoblastoma is the most common primary liver tumor of young children. There is an association with premature birth, such that the lower the birth weight, the higher the risk of hepatoblastoma.

▶ Patients with Beckwith-Wiedemann syndrome are at increased risk of developing hepatoblastoma, as well as Wilms' tumor, and are screened with ultrasound of the abdomen every 6 months throughout early childhood.

▶ Greater than 90% of hepatoblastomas are associated with markedly elevated levels of serum alpha-fetoprotein (AFP). The only other primary hepatic tumor of childhood associated with elevated AFP levels is hepatoma, which occurs in older children often with underlying hepatic disease.

▶ Hepatoblastoma generally appears as a very large, solid liver mass. Calcifications are visible in 15% of cases on CT. The tumor often appears lobulated. Central hemorrhage and necrosis are common. The tumor may invade hepatic or portal veins and most commonly spreads to adjacent lymph nodes and lung.

Next steps in management

Imaging evaluation for metastatic disease includes CT of the chest. Treatment is surgical resection. Neoadjuvant chemotherapy may render an unresectable tumor resectable and may decrease the extent of resection for a resectable tumor.

Further reading

1. Stocker JT. Hepatic tumors in children. Clin Liver Dis 2001;5:259–281, viii–ix.
2. Siegel MJ, Chung EM, Conran RM. Pediatric liver: focal masses. Magn Reson Imaging Clin North Am 2008;16:437–452, v.

History

► 8-week-old girl with lower-extremity flaccidity.

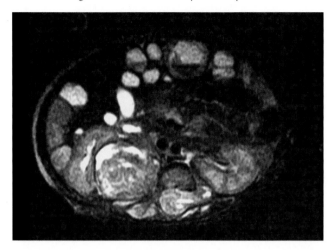

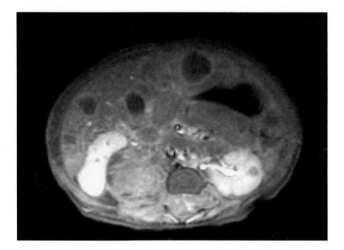

Case 16   Hepatic Metastases from Neuroblastoma

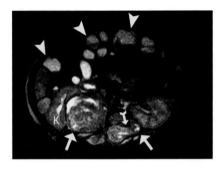 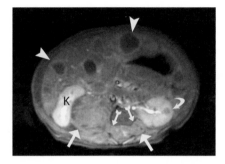

Findings

▸ Axial T2-weighted (left) and post-gadolinium T1-weighted (right) images show multiple liver masses (arrowheads) that are heterogeneous in signal intensity on T2, with fluid levels in some, and that show only rim enhancement on post-contrast images. Also seen are paraspinous masses (arrows) that extend through the neural foramina (tailed arrows) into the spinal canal. The right paraspinous mass displaces the right kidney (K) laterally.
A small lesion is noted in the left kidney (curved) arrow.

Differential diagnosis

The most common liver tumor in children, as in adults, is metastatic disease, particularly in cases of multiple lesions, and neuroblastoma is the most frequent primary tumor in this age group. The additional findings of bilateral paraspinous masses with extension into the spinal canal indicate the diagnosis of neuroblastoma. Multicentric infantile hemangioendothelioma (IHE) would be included in the differential diagnosis of the liver lesions. The imaging features of the hepatic lesions in this case are not consistent with IHE, however, in that the masses exhibit only rim enhancement, while IHE demonstrates intense peripheral nodular enhancement with centripetal fill-in.

Teaching points

▸ Multiple liver lesions usually represent metastatic disease. Other considerations include IHE and the rare angiosarcoma, which should be suspected in children who present after age 1 year or in children whose lesions do not respond to therapy for IHE.
▸ Common primary tumors causing liver metastases in children include neuroblastoma, which can be congenital, Wilms' tumor (usually late in the disease), and lymphoma. Lymphoma usually occurs in school-age or older children and the lesions may appear cystic on ultrasound.

Next steps in management

Tissue and bone marrow biopsy and evaluation for excess urinary catecholamines are the next steps, followed by chemotherapy.

Further reading

1. Lonergan GJ, Schwab CM, Suarez ES, Carlson CL. Neuroblastoma, ganglioneuroblastoma, and ganglioneuroma: radiologic-pathologic correlation. Radiographics. 2002 Jul–Aug;22(4):911–934.
2. Forman HP, Leonidas JC, Berdon WE, et al. Congenital neuroblastoma: evaluation with multimodality imaging. Radiology. 1990 May;175(2):365–368.

History

▶ 1-week-old premature infant with abdominal distention.

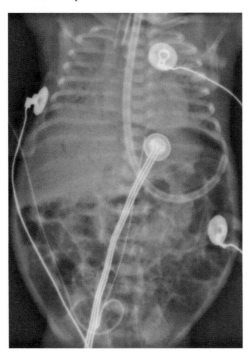

Case 17 Free Intraperitoneal Air with Necrotizing Enterocolitis

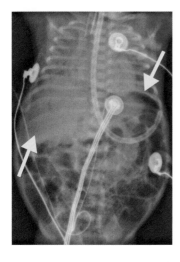 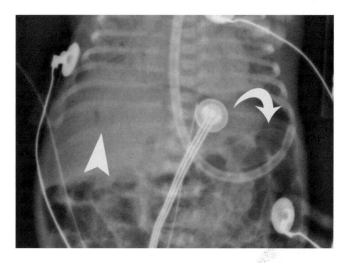

Findings

▶ Supine plain radiograph of the abdomen (left) demonstrates diffusely dilated loops of bowel and abnormal lucency over the liver and left upper quadrant under the diaphragm (arrows).

▶ Magnified view of the same radiograph (right) reveals both sides of the bowel wall (Rigler sign) indicating the presence of free air (curved arrow). Note the branched lucencies over the liver (arrowhead) representing portal venous gas due to necrotizing enterocolitis (NEC).

Differential diagnosis

In neonates, the most common cause of free intraperitoneal air is NEC with perforation. Spontaneous intestinal perforation in preterm infants without findings of NEC may also occur.

Teaching points

▶ Supine radiographs are insensitive for the finding of free intraperitoneal air, but sick premature infants are sensitive to positional changes, so decubitus or upright views are not routinely obtained. Findings of free air on the supine view include increased lucency over the abdomen with visualization of the falciform ligament surrounded by air ("football" sign) and air on both sides of the bowel wall in the absence of adjacent bowel loop (Rigler sign). Cross-table lateral views are sensitive for free air and do not require repositioning of the infant.

Next steps in management

Free intraperitoneal air is always an indication for surgical intervention. If the premature infant is too sick to withstand open surgery, placement of peritoneal drains in the NICU is an option.

Further reading

1. Buonomo C. The radiology of necrotizing enterocolitis. Radiol Clin North Am. 1999 Nov;37(6):1187–1198.
2. Pumberger W, et al. Spontaneous localized intestinal perforation in very-low-birth-weight infants: a distinct clinical entity different from necrotizing enterocolitis. J Am Coll Surg. 2002 Dec;195(6):796–803.

History

▶ 2-year-old on broad-spectrum antibiotic therapy with new abdominal pain.

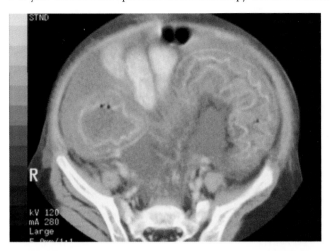

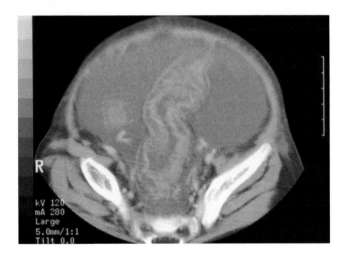

Case 18 *Clostridium difficile* Colitis

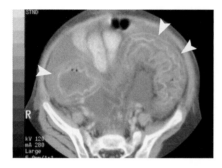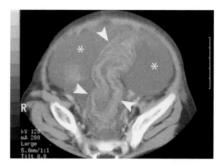

Findings

▶ Both CT images demonstrate marked, diffuse colonic wall thickening (arrowheads) with densely enhancing mucosa and serosa. The colonic lumen is fluid-filled. Additionally, moderate ascites is noted (asterisks).

Differential diagnosis

The finding of bowel wall thickening is very abnormal but not very specific, as it may also be caused by infection (salmonella, cytomegalivirus, Yersinia, tuberculosis, neutropenic enterocolitis), noninfectious inflammatory diseases (Crohn disease or ulcerative colitis, Henoch-Schönlein purpura, hemolytic uremic syndrome), neoplasm (leukemia or lymphoma), or ischemia/hypotension. The findings of marked colonic wall thickening and ascites in a patient on antibiotic therapy suggests the diagnosis of *C. difficile* colitis.

Teaching points

▶ *C. difficile* or pseudomembranous colitis is a complication of broad-spectrum antibiotic therapy or chemotherapy in which the gram-positive organism replaces the normal colonic flora and causes an infection. This complication has been reported with all antibiotics except vancomycin.

▶ The clinical spectrum of *C. difficile* colitis is quite variable and may be mild or may result in transmural necrosis and perforation.

▶ On CT the bowel mucosa enhances and appears quite dense adjacent to the edematous submucosa. Seen in the transverse plane, this appearance produces the "target" sign. If there is oral contrast in the affected bowel, the "accordion" sign may be observed. Pericolic stranding and ascites are also common findings. Ascites may be seen in other infectious colitides but is not typical of inflammatory bowel disease or neutropenic enterocolitis.

▶ Reduction of radiation dose is desirable and abdominal ultrasound should be considered in the evaluation of suspected colitis in children, as many of the above findings can also be demonstrated with ultrasound.

Next steps in management

The diagnosis is confirmed by demonstration of *C. difficile* toxin in the stool. Treatment is oral vancomycin or metronidazole.

Further reading

1. Kawamoto S, Horton KM, Fishman EK. Pseudomembranous colitis: spectrum of imaging findings with clinical and pathological correlation. Radiographics. 1999 Jul–Aug;19(4):887–897.
2. Cronin CG, O'Connor M, Lohan DG, et al. Imaging of the gastrointestinal complications of systemic chemotherapy. Clin Radiol. 2009 Jul;64(7):724–733.

History

▶ Newborn with imperforate anus. Choked with first feed.

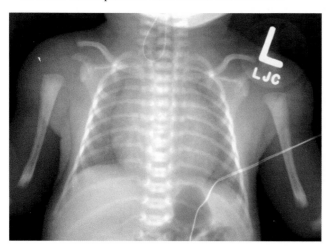

Case 19   Esophageal Atresia/VACTERL Association

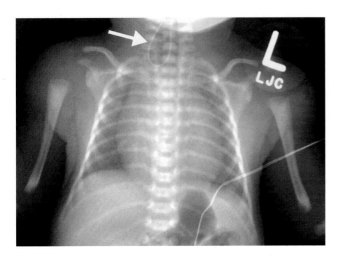

Findings

▶ AP view of the chest reveals an enteric tube coiled in the proximal esophageal pouch (arrow). Distal bowel gas is noted. The heart is enlarged.

Differential diagnosis

Inability to pass the enteric tube beyond the proximal third of the esophagus is a specific finding for esophageal atresia in a newborn.

Teaching points

▶ Esophageal atresia is part of a spectrum of incomplete separation of the foregut into the trachea and the esophagus. Frequently, there is a tracheo-esophageal (TE) fistula. Ninety-five percent of patients present in the first day of life.

▶ There are five types. In the most common type (82%), there is a fistula between the trachea and the distal esophagus allowing air into the distal bowel. The next most common type (8%) has no TE fistula. The third most common (6%) is the H-type fistula with intact esophagus.

▶ On prenatal imaging, polyhydramnios is observed. Only the minority of patients without a distal fistula have the specific finding of absence of the stomach bubble.

▶ TE fistula with esophageal atresia is part of the VACTERL association, which also includes vertebral anomalies, anal atresia, cardiac anomalies, and renal and limb anomalies. Diagnosis of esophageal atresia should prompt a search for other findings of the VACTERL association. The side of the aortic arch should be determined, if possible, on the chest radiograph. The surgeon will repair the esophagus through a thoracotomy on the side opposite that of the aortic arch. Cardiac anomalies, which are associated with right aortic arch, may be part of the VACTERL association.

▶ Further imaging with an esophagram is not necessary and will likely cause contrast aspiration. If the surgeon insists on further imaging, air can be safely injected through the enteric tube into the proximal pouch to distend it.

Next steps in management

Esophageal atresia is repaired surgically.

Further Reading

1. Buonomo C. Neonatal gastrointestinal emergencies. Radiol Clin North Am. 1997 Jul;35(4):845–864.
2. Berrocal T, Madrid C., Novo S, et al. Congenital anomalies of the tracheobronchial tree, lung and mediastinum: embryology, radiology, and pathology. Radiographics 2003;24:e17–e62.

History

► 6-year-old boy with dysphagia.

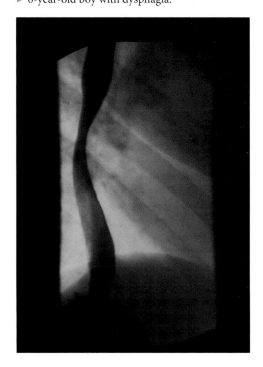

Case 20 Eosinophilic Esophagitis

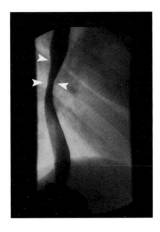

Findings

▸ Single-phase esophagram demonstrates a long tapered narrowing of the mid-esophagus (arrowheads).

Differential diagnosis

The differential diagnosis of a mid-esophageal narrowing also includes congenital causes (extrinsic compression from vascular ring or esophageal duplication cyst, intrinsic congenital esophageal stenosis), post-traumatic causes (caustic or disk battery ingestion, stricture after esophageal atresia repair), and infectious/inflammatory causes (candidiasis, cytomegalovirus, Barrett esophagus, Behçet disease, Crohn disease, epidermolysis bullosa, radiation therapy, and graft-versus-host disease). All of these appear similar radiographically, but clinical and laboratory data help to narrow the differential. Some radiographic findings are suggestive of certain diagnoses. Vascular rings cause smooth esophageal impressions at specific locations. Congenital esophageal stenosis may be associated with a ringed appearance, as can eosinophilic esophagitis. Infectious etiologies often cause marked mucosal irregularities. Peptic strictures most commonly involve the distal esophagus.

Teaching points

▸ Eosinophilic esophagitis is an idiopathic eosinophilic infiltration of the esophagus associated with a history of allergies and/or asthma. A marked male predominance has been noted.

▸ Patients present with symptoms of gastroesophageal reflux unresponsive to standard therapies, dysphagia, or food impaction.

▸ The esophagram is a relatively insensitive exam and most commonly appears normal in patients with eosinophilic esophagitis. The reason may be that the dysphagia is due to dysmotility rather than stricture. The most commonly observed abnormality of the esophagram is a long-segment narrowing in the mid- or distal esophagus. Mild mucosal irregularity may be observed but ulcerations are not seen. The finding of multiple distal esophageal ring-like narrowings is less common.

▸ Eosinophilic gastroenteritis may accompany esophagitis, but this is not common in children.

Next steps in management

Diagnosis is confirmed with endoscopy and biopsy. The condition is treated with institution of an elemental diet or with steroids.

Further reading

1. Binkovitz LA, Lorenz EA, Di Lorenzo C, Kahwash S. Pediatric eosinophilic esophagitis: radiologic findings with pathologic correlation. Pediatr Radiol. 2010 May;40(5):714–719.
2. Luedtke P, Levine MS, Rubesin SE, Weinstein DS, Laufer I. Radiologic diagnosis of benign esophageal strictures: a pattern approach. Radiographics. 2003 Jul–Aug;23(4):897–909.

History

▶ 2-month-old with nonprogressive, nonbilious emesis.

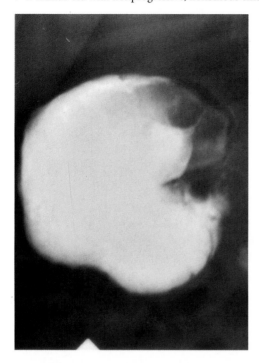

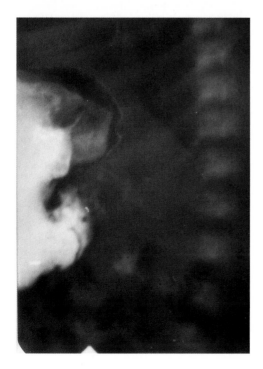

Case 21 Antral Web

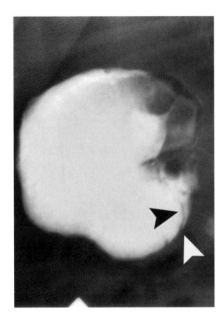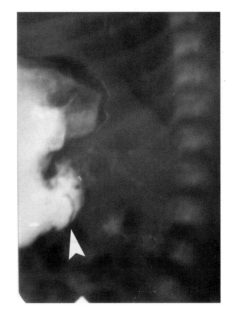

Findings

▶ Stair-step oblique images from an upper GI series show a curvilinear filling defect in the gastric antrum (arrowheads).

Differential diagnosis

The differential diagnosis for vomiting in an infant also includes hypertrophic pyloric stenosis (HPS) and gastroesophageal reflux (GER) for nonbilious emesis, and malrotation/midgut volvulus for bilious emesis. HPS is progressive while GER and antral web are not, but GER often resolves by age 1 year.

Teaching points

▶ Just as in other parts of the GI tract, the stomach can be congenitally obstructed due to atresia, stenosis, or web. Atresia is more common than stenosis or web and presents at birth with emesis after the first feed. Atresia is easy to diagnose; the stomach is dilated and there is no air beyond it, causing the single bubble appearance.

▶ The antral web has an opening, or fenestration, that allows passage of food and, consequently, has a more indolent presentation with nonprogressive, nonbilious emesis. The age at presentation depends on the size of the fenestration. Antral web is much more difficult to diagnose than gastric atresia, because the web is thin and surrounded by contrast on both sides. Stair-step oblique images or compression with the balloon to thin the contrast may be necessary to visualize the web.

Next steps in management

Antral web is treated surgically.

Further reading

1. Buonomo C. Neonatal gastrointestinal emergencies. Radiol Clin North Am. 1997 Jul;35(4):845–864.
2. Berrocal T, Torres I, Gutiérrez J, et al. Cogenital anomalies of the upper gastrointestinal tract. Radiographics. 1999;19(4):855–872.

History

▶ 5-week-old with vomiting.

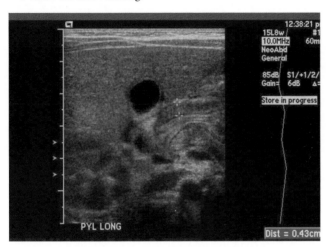

Case 22 Hypertrophic Pyloric Stenosis (HPS)

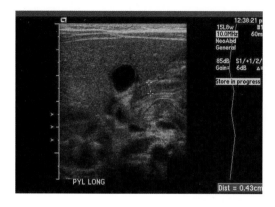 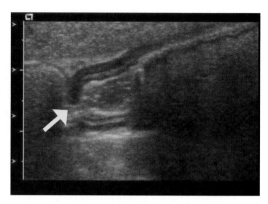

Findings

▶ Longitudinal image (left) shows a markedly elongated pylorus with muscle wall thickness (calipers) greater than 3 mm.

▶ Comparison image of a normal pylorus (arrow) reveals that the channel is very short, about 2 mm long, which is the same as the muscle thickness.

Differential diagnosis

Pylorospasm can mimic hypertrophic pyloric stenosis (HPS) in that the sphincter does not open, but the muscle wall is not thickened. A potential pitfall is the collapsed gastric antrum, which may be mistaken for an elongated pylorus, though the muscle wall is less than 3 mm thick. This pitfall can be avoided by turning the baby toward its right, so that the gastric fluid moves from the fundus to the antrum to distend it. If additional fluid is needed, electrolyte solution or glucose water may be given.

Teaching points

▶ HPS is an acquired rather than a congenital condition, although the etiology is unknown. HPS has a characteristic natural history that limits the age at presentation to 2 to 9 weeks. Symptoms develop and become progressively worse, causing dehydration, so that HPS is rare after age 3 months.

▶ Because the obstruction is proximal to the ampulla of Vater, the emesis is nonbilious. With bilious emesis an urgent upper GI series is indicated.

▶ Pyloric ultrasound in HPS shows an elongated antropyloric channel (14 mm or more) and the muscle wall thickness, as measured on one side from the echogenic mucosa to the echogenic serosa, is greater than 3 mm. If the pylorus is elongated and does not open yet is less than or equal to 3 mm, the exam may be repeated the following day, as HPS will get worse.

▶ If the pylorus is normal on the ultrasound, the superior mesenteric artery/vein relationship should be determined.

Next steps in management

In the U.S., the treatment is surgical pyloromyotomy. In some countries, nonoperative management is preferred.

Further reading

1. Hernanz-Schulman M. Infantile hypertrophic pyloric stenosis. Radiology. 2003 May;227(2):319–331.
2. Vasavada P. Ultrasound evaluation of acute abdominal emergencies. Radiol Clin North Am. 2004 Mar;42(2):445.

History

▶ 6-week-old with emesis and normal pyloric ultrasound. Second image from another patient.

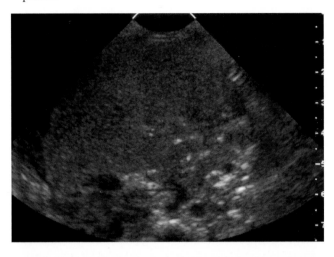

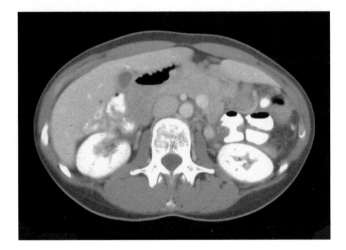

Case 23   Inversion of SMA and SMV in Malrotation

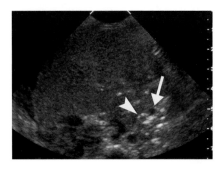
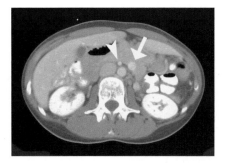

Findings

▶ Transverse ultrasound image (left) shows that the superior mesenteric vein (SMV) (arrow) is located to the left of the superior mesenteric artery (SMA) (arrowhead). An urgent upper GI series showed malrotation.

▶ CT image of an older patient shows the same finding of the SMV (arrow) located to the left of the SMA (arrowhead).

Differential diagnosis

The imaging differential diagnosis for emesis in a young infant depends on the character of the emesis. Bilious emesis suggests an obstruction distal to the ampulla of Vater. The diagnosis that must be excluded is midgut volvulus.

Teaching points

▶ Malrotation is a congenital anomaly of the development of the midgut. During weeks 5 to 6 of gestation, the midgut herniates into the umbilical cord and normally rotates 270 degrees counterclockwise before returning to the abdomen with the jejunum in the left upper quadrant and the cecum in the right lower quadrant. These loops of bowel form the ends of the root of the mesentery and they are normally widely separated, so that the bowel is stable in fixation. Abnormal rotation of the midgut causes malfixation of the bowel such that the ends of the root of the mesentery are close together. This allows the bowel to pivot around this narrow point of fixation, potentially causing midgut volvulus.

▶ Normally the SMV is on the right side of the SMA as it joins the splenic vein to form the portal vein. The finding of inversion of the SMA and SMV relationship has a high association with malrotation, but evaluation of the SMA/SMV relationship is not a good screening study for malrotation, since approximately one third of patients with surgically proven malrotation have a normal SMA/SMV relationship.

Next steps in management

An urgent upper GI series is indicated.

Further reading

1. Strouse PJ. Disorders of intestinal rotation and fixation ("malrotation"). Pediatr Radiol 2004;34:837–851.
2. Zerin JM, DiPietro MA. Superior mesenteric vascular anatomy at ultrasound in patients with surgically proved malrotation of the midgut. Radiology 1992;183:693–694.

History

▶ 2-day-old with emesis.

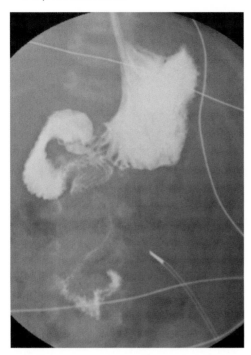

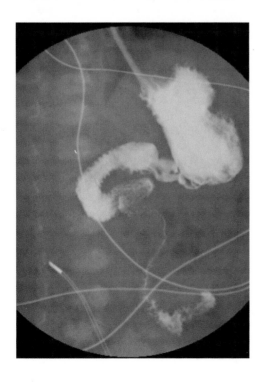

Case 24 Midgut Volvulus

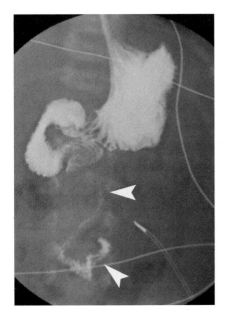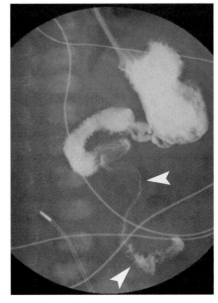

Findings

▶ AP (left) and lateral (right) images from an upper GI series demonstrate an abnormal corkscrew course of the jejunum (arrowheads).

Differential diagnosis

This finding is diagnostic.

Teaching points

▶ Patients with midgut volvulus are predisposed by malrotation and malfixation of the bowel during embryonic life.
▶ The vast majority of patients with midgut volvulus present in the first month of life with a catastrophic course. Although delayed presentation is less common, midgut volvulus must be considered in any child with bilious emesis. In patients who present in early infancy, the root of the mesentery is very narrow and the bowel twists more than 360 degrees so that the arterial supply from the superior mesenteric artery is occluded. In patients who present later, the root of the mesentery is narrower than normal but not severely narrow. Volvulus may be partial and intermittent, occluding the venous drainage but not the arterial supply, leading to bowel wall thickening, malabsorption, and diarrhea. Catastrophic volvulus can occur in these patients too.
▶ Imaging should begin with a KUB to exclude distal obstruction, which also causes bilious emesis. The classic appearance for midgut volvulus is obstruction of the second or third portion of the duodenum. Most often the KUB is normal, a finding that should not dissuade one from performing an upper GI series. In fact, in a newborn, midgut volvulus is the only cause of obstruction that produces a normal plain film.
▶ In any infant, any duodenal obstruction is an indication for emergent surgery. More specific findings of midgut volvulus (beak or the corkscrew) are not necessary to go to surgery.

Next steps in management

The treatment for midgut volvulus is an emergent Ladd procedure, at the conclusion of which all the small bowel is on the right and all the large bowel is on the left.

Further reading

1. Buonomo C. Neonatal gastrointestinal emergencies. Radiol Clin North Am 1997;35:845–864.
2. Shew SB. Surgical concerns in malrotation and midgut volvulus. Pediatr Radiol 2009;30 Suppl 2:S167–S171.

History

► Newborn with bilious emesis.

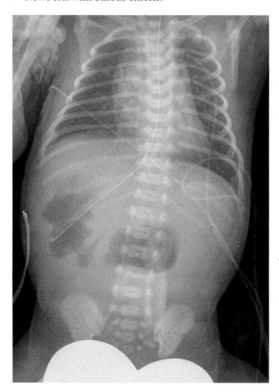

Case 25   Duodenal Atresia and Heterotaxy

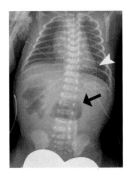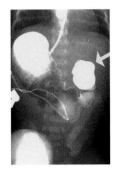

Findings

▶ Supine radiograph of the abdomen shows an enteric tube with the tip in the stomach, which is on the opposite side of the cardiac apex (arrowhead), indicating heterotaxy. The duodenal bulb is dilated (arrow) and there is no distal bowel gas. This is the "double bubble" sign of duodenal atresia.

▶ The true double bubble with complete obstruction is diagnostic and no further imaging is required. An upper GI series was performed and confirmed duodenal atresia in this patient with heterotaxy.

Differential diagnosis

If the duodenal bulb is dilated but there is distal bowel gas, then two entities must be considered in the differential diagnosis—duodenal stenosis and midgut volvulus. Both are surgical, but if surgery is not immediate, an urgent upper GI series is indicated in the case of partial obstruction of the duodenum to rule out midgut volvulus.

Teaching points

▶ Duodenal atresia is thought to be due to failure of canalization of the foregut, which begins as a solid cord of cells. Atresia is more common than stenosis or web.

▶ About 30% of patients with duodenal atresia have Down syndrome. Duodenal atresia/stenosis is also associated with annular pancreas, preduodenal portal vein, other GI atresias, biliary anomalies, congenital heart disease, and VACTERL.

▶ The obstruction is almost always distal to the ampulla of Vater so that the patient has bilious emesis.

▶ Polyhydramnios and the sonolucent double bubble sign are observed on prenatal ultrasound in duodenal atresia. The finding of the double bubble in utero should prompt evaluation for chromosomal disorders.

▶ The duodenal web is fenestrated and if the opening is large, presentation may be delayed until adulthood. Over time, peristalsis causes elongation of the web and the "windsock deformity," also known as intraduodenal diverticulum. This diverticulum may obstruct the biliary or pancreatic ducts.

Next steps in management

The treatment for duodenal atresia is surgical repair.

Further reading

1. Buonomo C. Neonatal gastrointestinal emergencies. Radiol Clin North Am. 1997 Jul;35(4):845–864.
2. Berrocal T, Torres I, Gutiérrez J, et al. Congenital anomalies of the upper gastrointestinal tract. Radiographics.1999;19(4):855–872.

History

▶ Newborn with abdominal distention and bilious emesis.

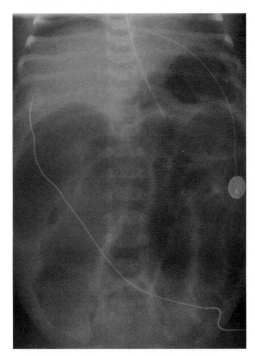

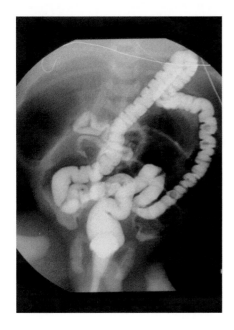

Case 26   Ileal Atresia

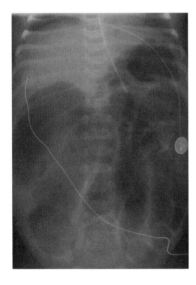 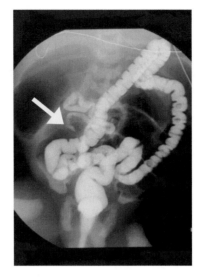

Findings

▶ The supine radiograph of the abdomen (left) demonstrates multiple, dilated tubular loops of bowel indicating distal obstruction.

▶ The contrast enema (right) shows a microcolon and abrupt termination of the contrast column at the site of bowel discontinuity in the ileum (arrow) with no contrast filling of the air-filled, dilated proximal bowel.

Differential diagnosis

The differential diagnosis of distal bowel obstruction in the newborn also includes meconium ileus, colonic atresia, functional immaturity of the colon, and Hirschsprung disease. The finding of complete microcolon on contrast enema narrows the differential diagnosis to ileal atresia and meconium ileus. Contrast must be refluxed into the ileum to distinguish the two. There is abrupt cut-off of the contrast column in ileal atresia, while it is possible to reflux contrast past the obstruction into dilated proximal bowel in meconium ileus.

Teaching points

▶ Any bowel obstruction distal to the ampulla of Vater can cause bilious emesis. Start the work-up of bilious emesis with a plain radiograph of the abdomen, which will differentiate proximal (few dilated bowel loops) from distal (many dilated loops) obstruction. Distal obstruction may be medical or surgical in origin.

▶ The next step is a contrast enema, which distinguishes medical from surgical causes and can be used to treat medical causes.

▶ In newborns, swallowed air may have not yet reached a site of perforation, so it is possible to have a bowel perforation without the finding of free air. Barium should not be used in the performance of the enema. Hyperosmolar contrast must also be avoided as it can draw fluid into the colon from the intravascular space and cause fatal electrolyte imbalances. High- or low-osmolar, water-soluble contrast agents can be diluted to the osmolality of serum (285 mOsm/kg of water).

Next steps in management

Ileal atresia is repaired surgically.

Further reading

1. Buonomo C. Neonatal gastrointestinal emergencies. Radiol Clin North Am. 1997 Jul;35(4):845–864.
2. Berrocal T, Lamas M, Gutieérrez J, et al. Congenital anomalies of the small intestine, colon, and rectum. Radiographics. 1999;19(5):1219–1236.

History

▶ Newborn with abdominal distention and failure to pass meconium. Parents are cystic fibrosis carriers.

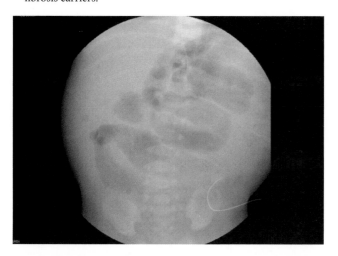

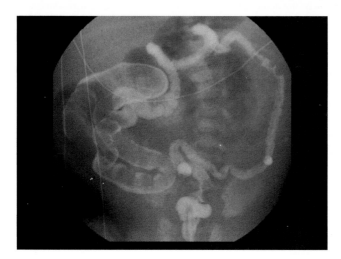

Case 27   Meconium Ileus in Infant with Cystic Fibrosis

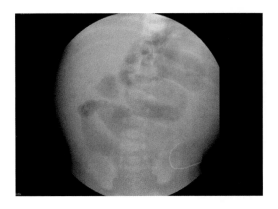 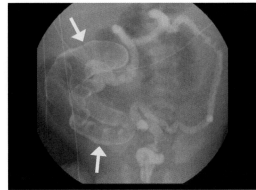

Findings

▶ The frontal scout radiograph (left) shows several dilated tubular loops of bowel indicating distal obstruction.

▶ Frontal view from a contrast enema reveals a microcolon and large filling defects in the small bowel (arrows).

Differential diagnosis

Other causes of distal bowel obstruction in the neonate include medical and surgical lesions, and contrast enema is indicated to differentiate these. Both meconium ileus and ileal atresia are associated with microcolon (less than 1 cm in diameter). In meconium ileus, the bowel is intact but the meconium is abnormally thick and inspissated, forming obstructing filling defects in the distal ileum. Normally, there is no solid material in the small bowel. Also, if contrast is refluxed beyond the obstruction, dilated proximal small bowel will be opacified.

Teaching points

▶ Virtually all infants with meconium ileus have cystic fibrosis, and neonatal GI obstruction is the presenting sign in 5% to 20% of patients with cystic fibrosis.

▶ Suggestive radiographic findings include a soap-bubble appearance of meconium mixed with air in the right lower quadrant with absence of air–fluid levels on cross-table radiographs.

▶ Approximately half of infants with meconium ileus can be treated medically. The rest develop complications that necessitate surgery. Complications include volvulus around the mass of retained meconium, bowel necrosis, and perforation.

Next steps in management

Hyperosmolar contrast can draw fluid into the bowel and loosen the meconium, so that the enema is therapeutic as well as diagnostic. The enema may be repeated once or twice daily as long as the infant continues to clinically improve. If there is no clinical improvement, a complication should be suspected and surgery considered.

Further reading

1. Kao SC, et al. Nonoperative treatment of simple meconium ileus: a survey of the Society for Pediatric Radiology. Pediatr Radiol 1987;162:447–456.
2. Berrocal T, Lammas M, Gutieerez J, et al. Congenital anomalies of the small intestine, colon, and rectum. Radiographics 1999 Sep–Oct;19(5):1219–1236.

History

▸ 7-year-old girl with 1 week of intermittent abdominal pain and vomiting.

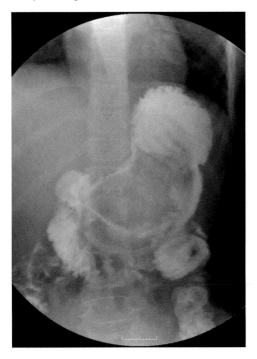

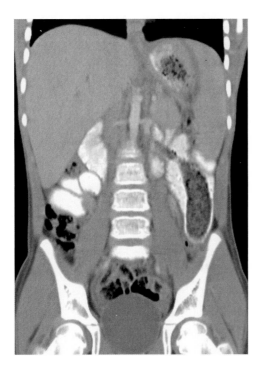

Case 28 Embolic Trichobezoar

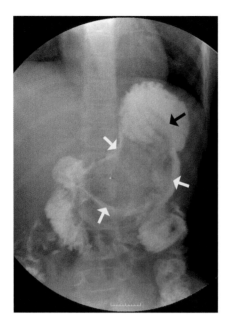 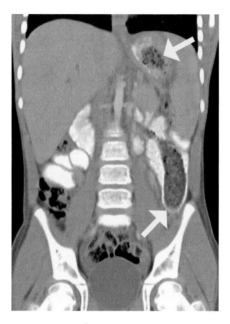

Findings

▶ Frontal view from an upper GI series (left) shows a large filling defect in the stomach (arrows).
▶ On the coronal CT image (right), a mottled gastric filling defect is seen as well as a similar tubular filling defect in the jejunum (arrows).

Differential diagnosis

If the filling defect is limited to the stomach, undigested food should also be considered. This patient had not eaten in many hours.

Teaching points

▶ In adults, bezoars are commonly composed of undigested plant materials or pills and are frequently related to prior surgery causing stasis. In children, on the other hand, bezoars are commonly composed of undissolved formula (lactobezoar) or ingested hair (trichobezoar).
▶ Clues to the presence of a trichobezoar may include an area of alopecia on the same side as the dominant hand or absence of hair on a favorite doll.
▶ Trichobezoars may become embolic with smaller, distal hairballs attached to the gastric hairball by strands of hair.

Next steps in management

Lactobezoars are treated by adding water to the formula. Trichobezoars can be treated endoscopically as long as they are not embolic. Embolic bezoars require surgical treatment.

Further reading

1. Malhotra A, Jones L, Drugas G. Simultaneous gastric and small intestinal trichobezoars. Pediatr Emerg Care 2008 Nov;24(11):774–776.

History

▶ Newborn with prenatal ultrasound finding.

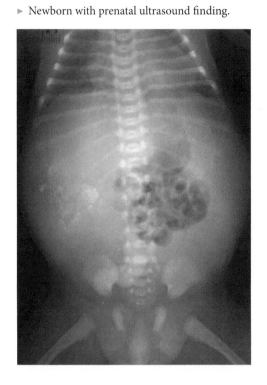

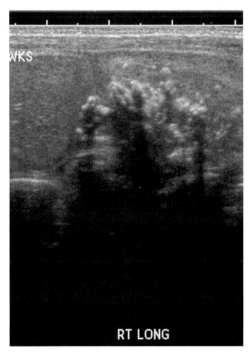

Case 29 Meconium Peritonitis

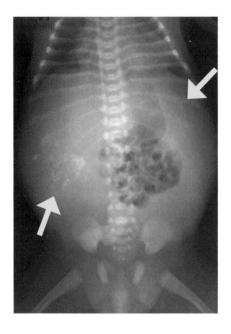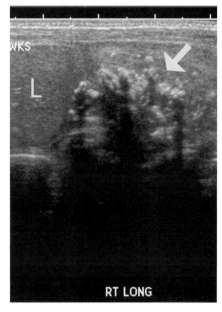

Findings

▶ Supine plain radiograph (left) demonstrates clustered amorphous calcifications in both upper quadrants (arrows).

▶ Longitudinal ultrasound image shows a cluster of shadowing echogenic foci (arrow) adjacent to the liver (L).

Differential diagnosis

The finding of abdominal calcification indicates meconium peritonitis, but the underlying cause may be meconium ileus, bowel atresia, or in utero volvulus. In half of cases, no cause is found at birth.

Teaching points

▶ Meconium peritonitis is due to in utero perforation of bowel with leakage of meconium into the peritoneal cavity with subsequent inflammatory reaction and calcification. Frequently, the perforation has sealed by the time the infant is born.

▶ Depending on the distribution of the meconium, meconium peritonitis may take several forms. The calcification may appear linear, in clusters, or may be localized to the periphery of a mass (meconium pseudocyst). The distribution may be generalized, frequently found under the hemidiaphragms or in the paracolic gutters. In boys, the meconium may pass through the patent processus vaginalis to the scrotum (meconium periorchitis).

Next steps in management

If the infant has obstructive symptoms, plain radiography may reveal evidence of upper or lower obstruction. Upper GI obstruction in infants is always surgical. If there is evidence of lower GI obstruction, then contrast enema is indicated.

Further reading

1. Buonomo C. Neonatal gastrointestinal emergencies. Radiol Clin North Am. 1997 Jul;35(4):845–864.
2. Berrocal T, Lammas M, Gutieerez J, et al. Congenital anomalies of the small intestine, colon, and rectum. Radiographics 1999 Sep–Oct;19(5):1219–1236.

History

▶ 1-month-old girl with bilious emesis.

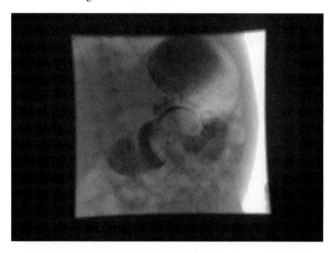

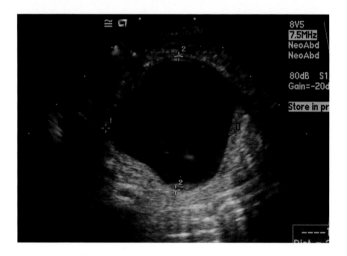

Case 30   Duodenal Duplication Cyst

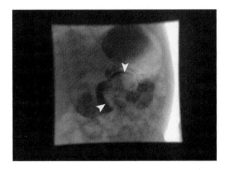
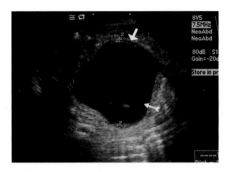

Findings

▶ Oblique image from an upper GI series (left) shows dilation of the third portion of the duodenum with a well-circumscribed mural mass (arrowheads).

▶ Ultrasound image shows a cyst with multilaminar wall ("gut signature") (arrow) and internal echoes representing debris (tailed arrow).

Differential diagnosis

Other cystic lesions in this location include choledochal cyst, lymphatic malformation, pancreatic cyst, and mature cystic teratoma. The finding of "gut signature" of the wall on ultrasound and the unilocular appearance suggest a duplication cyst.

Teaching points

▶ Enteric duplication cysts are developmental anomalies on the mesenteric side of the GI tract. They can occur anywhere along the GI tract and are named for the adjacent bowel with which they share a wall and blood supply. They are usually round and do not communicate with the bowel lumen, although they may be tubular and communicate with the bowel lumen, particularly in the colon. Duplication cysts most commonly arise in the ileum (40%) followed by the thorax.

▶ Clinical presentation—Many are diagnosed prenatally. Because most do not communicate with the adjacent bowel lumen, they accumulate succus entericus and enlarge, eventually causing obstructive symptoms. Additionally, like Meckel diverticulum, duplication cysts may contain heterotopic gastric mucosa or pancreatic tissue. Intralesional hemorrhage may lead to an acute presentation with abdominal pain.

▶ Ultrasound is the preferred exam for diagnosis. The "rim" sign of gut signature in the wall is most helpful. Additionally, peristalsis is observed in the cyst during real-time examination. Echogenic internal debris from prior hemorrhage or infection may be noted.

Next steps in management

Duplication cysts are treated with surgical resection.

Further reading

1. Berrocal T, Torres I, Gutiérrez J, et al. Congenital anomalies of the upper gastrointestinal tract. Radiographics. 1999 Jul–Aug;19(4):855–872.

2. Wootton-Gorges SL, Thomas KB, Harned RK, et al. Giant cystic abdominal masses in children. Pediatr Radiol. 2005 Dec;35(12):1277–1288.

History

▶ 6-year-old boy with abdominal pain after playing soccer.

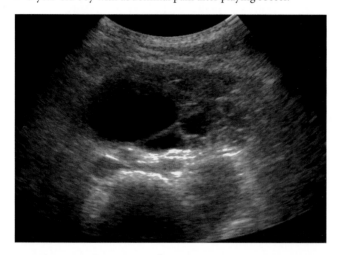

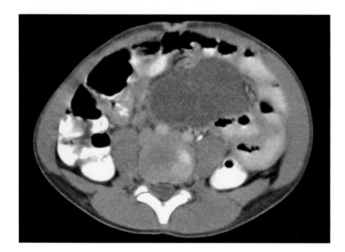

Case 31 Mesenteric Lymphangioma (Lymphatic Malformation)

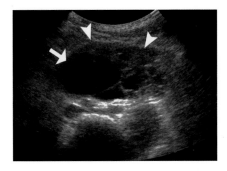 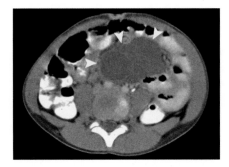

Findings

▶ Transverse ultrasound image (left) reveals a mass (arrowheads) anterior to the bifurcation of the aorta that is predominantly cystic (arrow).

▶ Axial CT image (right) demonstrates a predominantly cystic mass (arrowheads) displacing bowel loops anteriorly.

Differential diagnosis

Other cystic lesions in the pediatric abdomen include enteric duplication cyst, mesenteric or omental cyst, ureteropelvic junction obstruction, multicystic dysplastic kidney, choledochal cyst, ovarian cyst or chronic torsion, and mature cystic teratoma. The lymphangioma or lymphatic malformation is ovoid or lobulated and multilocular and does not demonstrate gut signature in its wall.

Teaching points

▶ Lymphangiomas, or lymphatic malformations, are the result of abnormal development of lymph channels. Most occur in the neck, superior mediastinum, and axilla, but they uncommonly arise in the mesentery, omentum, or retroperitoneum.

▶ Clinical presentation is variable. Patients may present with an asymptomatic mass, pain, obstructive symptoms, or even acute abdomen due to bowel volvulus or intralesional hemorrhage.

▶ Plain radiographs usually show a soft-tissue density displacing bowel loops. Bowel loops may appear dilated if the cyst is causing obstruction. On imaging, the malformation most commonly appears as a multilocular macrocystic mass, but microcystic portions may appear solid. The fluid appears homogenous on CT but may contain internal echoes on US. The mass is intimately associated with bowel and displaces it. The mass may completely surround a loop of bowel. In complicated cases, dilated bowel loops or the "swirl" or "whirlpool" sign" of volvulus may be noted.

Next steps in management

If discovered on ultrasound, CT or MR is the next step to determine the relationship to other organs and to help diagnose complications. Treatment is complete surgical excision of the cyst and, if necessary, involved portions of bowel.

Further reading

1. Traubici J, Daneman A, Wales P, et al. Mesenteric lymphatic malformation associated with small bowel volvulus—two cases and a review of the literature. Pediatr Radiol. 2002;32:362–365.
2. Konen O, Rathaus V, Dlugy E, et al. Childhood abdominal cystic lymphangioma. Pediatr Radiol. 2002;32:88–94.

History

▶ 3-year-old girl with colicky abdominal pain.

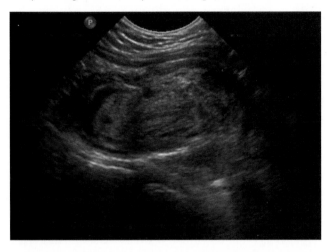

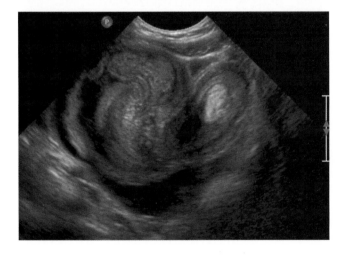

Case 32   Meckel Diverticulum Causing Ileocolic Intussusception

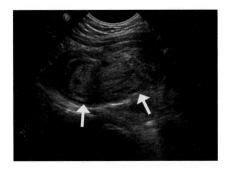 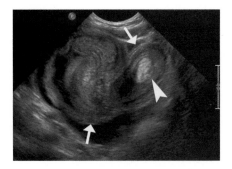

Findings

▶ Oblique ultrasound images show the multi-layered appearance of bowel within bowel (arrows) with a central echogenic tubular structure (arrowhead), representing mesenteric fat within an inverted Meckel diverticulum.

Differential diagnosis

The differential diagnosis of abdominal pain includes intussusception, obstruction due to hernia, appendicitis, torsed ovary, and pyelonephritis. Abdominal ultrasound can be used to diagnose any of these in a young child.

Teaching points

▶ Meckel diverticulum is a remnant of the omphalomesenteric or vitelline duct and the most common congenital GI anomaly.

▶ Rule of 2's—occurs in about 2% of the population, within 2 feet of the ileocecal valve, and is around 2 inches long. Approximately 2% of patients present with complications, usually by age 2 years.

▶ Complications include bleeding, which is the most common, and diverticulitis. The diverticulum may also invert and serve as the lead point for an intussusception, causing obstruction. Obstruction is the second most common complication. Meckel diverticulum is the most common lead point causing intussusception in infants younger than 6 months of age.

▶ Meckel diverticulum is a true diverticulum that is found on the antimesenteric side of the ileum. Those found incidentally are usually lined with small-bowel epithelium, while those that cause bleeding or diverticulitis often contain heterotopic gastric mucosa or pancreatic tissue.

▶ In patients who present with painless lower GI bleeding, the Meckel scan, which uses free pertechnetate, will localize the site of heterotopic gastric mucosa in the right lower quadrant.

▶ For patients who present with obstructive symptoms rather than bleeding, ultrasound is very helpful, while the Meckel scan is likely to be negative due to absence of heterotopic gastric mucosa.

Next steps in management

Intussusception due to a lead point is treated surgically.

Further reading

1. Levy AD, Hobbs CM. From the archives of the AFIP. Meckel diverticulum: radiologic features with pathologic correlation. Radiographics. 2004 Mar–Apr;24(2):565–587.
2. Berrocal T, Lamas M, Gutiérrez J, et al. Congenital anomalies of the small intestine, colon, and rectum. Radiographics. 1999;19(5):1219–1236.

History

▶ 27-week fetus with a finding on routine prenatal ultrasound.

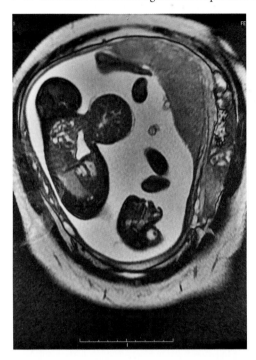

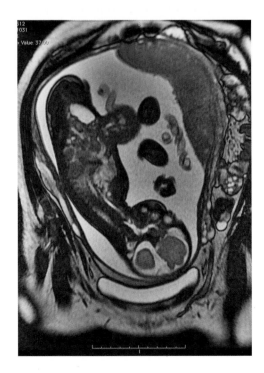

Case 33 Omphalocele

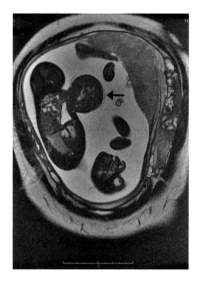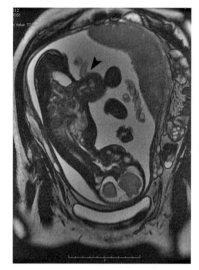

Findings

▶ Sagittal T2-weighted prenatal MR (left) shows liver outside the abdominal cavity surrounded by a thin membrane (arrow).

▶ Another sagittal image (right) shows the insertion of the cord into the hernia sac (arrowhead).

Differential diagnosis

▶ The differential diagnosis consists of other abdominal wall defects, particularly gastroschisis. Omphalocele represents a midline defect that allows herniation of bowel and/or liver into the base of the umbilical cord, so that the herniated organs are contained by a membrane of peritoneum, amnion, and Wharton's jelly. In contradistinction, gastroschisis is a full-thickness abdominal wall defect to the right of a normal cord insertion. The herniated material consists of bowel, which is freely floating in the amniotic fluid. Exposure to amniotic fluid often causes bowel wall thickening in gastroschisis. Additionally, the maternal serum alpha-fetoprotein level is elevated in gastroschisis but not omphalocele.

Teaching points

▶ Physiologically herniated bowel should return to the abdomen by 12 weeks' gestation.

▶ Omphalocele has a high association with other developmental anomalies as well as chromosomal anomalies and Beckwith-Wiedemann syndrome (omphalocele, macrosomia, and macroglossia). On the other hand, gastroschisis is almost always an isolated finding.

▶ The postoperative course is usually more complicated in gastroschisis compared to omphalocele, because the exposure to amniotic fluid may cause thickening of the bowel wall and hypoperistalsis.

Next steps in management

A search for other anomalies, especially cardiac anomalies, with ultrasound, cardiac echo, and possibly pre-natal MR, is the next step in evaluation of an infant with omphalocele. The overall prognosis depends on the presence and severity of associated anomalies. In the absence of other anomalies, the prognosis is quite good.

Further reading

1. Bair JH, Russ PD, Pretorius DH, et al. Fetal omphalocele and gastroschisis: a review of 24 cases. AJR Am J Roentgenol 1986;147:1047–1051.
2. Sugai Y, Hosoya T, Kurachi H. MR Imaging of fetal omphalocele. Magn Reson Med Sci. 2008;7(4):211–213.

History

▶ 2-week old with abdominal distention and emesis.

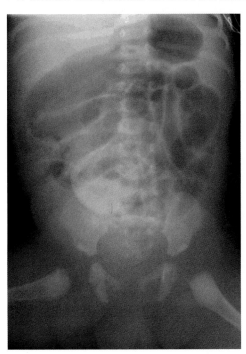

Case 34   Small Bowel Obstruction/Incarcerated Umbilical Hernia

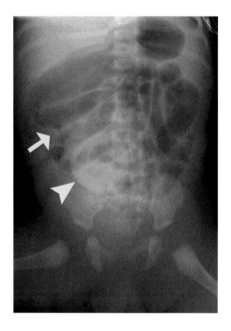 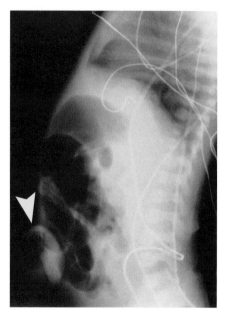

Findings

▶ AP (left) and lateral (right) radiographs demonstrate multiple dilated tubular loops of bowel (arrow) consistent with obstruction. Also noted is a sharply circumscribed soft-tissue density (arrowhead) representing an umbilical hernia surrounded by air, which is the cause of the obstruction.

Differential diagnosis

The most common cause of small bowel obstruction in adults is postsurgical adhesions, but these are uncommon in children. More common causes of bowel obstruction in infants and young children are intussusception and incarcerated hernias. Less common causes include midgut volvulus, Ladd bands, appendicitis, and tumors.

Teaching points

▶ Umbilical and inguinal hernias are very common in children. Umbilical hernias are clinically obvious and rarely become incarcerated, so they do not pose a diagnostic question for the radiologist.
▶ Inguinal hernias in children are indirect and 90% occur in boys. Premature infants have an increased risk. Inguinal hernias may become incarcerated and should be surgically repaired.
▶ Plain radiographic findings of inguinal hernia in a child include asymmetry of the inguinal folds and air projecting over the inguinal region on a supine radiograph.
▶ Sonography is the study of choice for suspected inguinal hernia. Bowel is the most common abdominal structure to herniate into the inguinal region, but mesenteric fat, ascitic fluid, and even ovaries can also herniate. Color Doppler interrogation of the wall of the herniated bowel is helpful for the surgeon.

Next steps in management

The treatment for bowel obstruction in children is surgical unless the obstruction is caused by an ileocolic intussusception in a child in the proper age group for idiopathic intussusception. In such a case, reduction by contrast enema may be attempted. The watchful waiting that is employed with adults is not appropriate for children.

Further reading

1. McCollough M, Sharieff GQ. Abdominal pain in children. Pediatr Clin North Am. 2006 Feb;53(1):107–137, vi.
2. Graf JL, Caty MG, Martin DJ, Glick PL. Pediatric hernias. Semin Ultrasound CT MR. 2002 Apr;23(2):197–200.

History

▶ 5-year-old with abdominal pain.

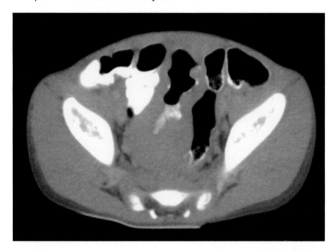

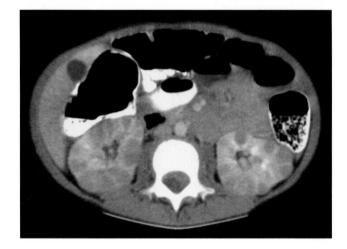

Case 35 Burkitt Lymphoma Involving Ileum and Kidneys

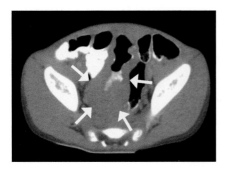 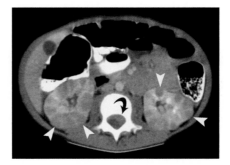

Findings

▶ CT image (left) shows circumferential bowel wall thickening with focal mass-like areas (arrows).

▶ More cephalad CT image demonstrates multiple, bilateral, hypoattenuating renal masses (arrowheads) and a mass in the spinal canal (curved arrow).

Differential diagnosis

The finding of bowel wall thickening has a broad differential, including infectious, inflammatory, neoplastic, and vascular causes. The presence of focal mass-like areas of thickening, the absence of inflammatory changes in the surrounding fat, and the presence of renal and other masses suggest Burkitt lymphoma.

Teaching points

▶ Burkitt lymphoma, a type of non-Hodgkin lymphoma, is the most common abdominal lymphoma in children and the fastest-growing pediatric tumor, with a doubling time of 24 hours.

▶ The World Health Organization recognizes three types.

  ▪ Endemic—found in equatorial Africa and Papua New Guinea, has a high association with Epstein-Barr virus infection, and often involves the head and neck

  ▪ Sporadic (American)—found in North America and Europe and commonly involves abdominal organs

  ▪ Immunodeficiency related—occurs in children with HIV/AIDS, allografts, or congenital immune disorders

▶ Burkitt lymphoma commonly involves the GI tract, especially the ileocecal region, and may cause diffuse mural thickening or focal masses. The latter are common lead points for intussusceptions in children over the age of 4 years. Cavitary lesions that communicate with the bowel lumen infrequently occur.

▶ Retroperitoneum and mesentery are potential sites of adenopathy. Solid organs are common sites of disease, including the kidneys, liver, spleen, pancreas, ovaries, and breasts.

Next steps in management

Imaging for staging commonly includes CT, PET/CT, bone scintigraphy, and gallium scanning. PET/CT provides more anatomic information than gallium scanning and is likely more sensitive. With the increased concern about cumulative radiation dose, MR is likely to become more important in diagnosis and follow-up. The treatment is chemotherapy.

Further reading

1. Abramson SJ, Price AP. Imaging of pediatric lymphomas. Radiol Clin North Am. 2008 Mar;46(2):313–338, ix.
2. Jadvar H, Connolly LP, Fahey FH, Shulkin BL. PET and PET/CT in pediatric oncology. Semin Nucl Med. 2007 Sep;37(5):316–331.

History

▶ 6-day-old premature infant.

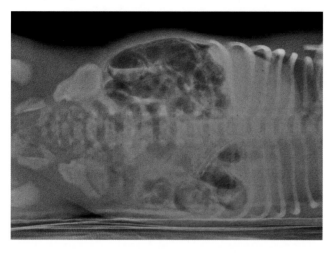

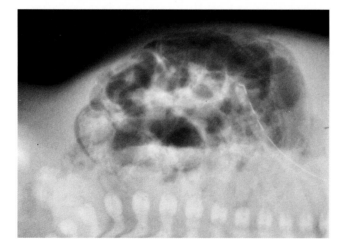

Case 36 Necrotizing Enterocolitis with Perforation

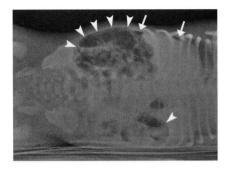 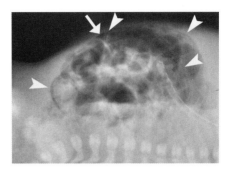

Findings

▶ Left lateral decubitus (left) and cross-table lateral (right) radiographs show extensive subserosal pneumatosis (curvilinear air lucency in the bowel wall [arrowheads]) and free intraperitoneal air (arrows).

Differential diagnosis

The finding of pneumatosis is usually not benign in children as it may be in adults. In premature infants, this is a specific finding of necrotizing enterocolitis (NEC). Pneumatosis may also be seen in neutropenic enterocolitis.

Teaching points

▶ Premature infants are at significant risk of developing NEC, but NEC can also occur in term infants with cyanotic congenital heart disease, Hirschsprung disease, or umbilical artery catheters.

▶ Nonspecific findings of NEC on radiographs include multiple dilated tubular loops of bowel due to ileus, thickened bowel wall, and ascites. An unchanging loop of bowel over the course of follow-up (the sentinel loop sign) is concerning for bowel necrosis.

▶ Specific findings of NEC include submucosal and subserosal pneumatosis. The former appears as mottled air lucency similar to stool. Portal venous gas is also specific for NEC.

▶ Subserosal pneumatosis, portal venous gas, and free air can also be detected with ultrasound, and follow-up studies can be performed with ultrasound, reducing radiation dose. Thinning of the bowel wall and lack of color Doppler flow are US findings that may precede free air on plain radiography.

▶ The major short-term complication is bowel perforation. Bowel stricture may be a long-term complication. Contrast enema can be used to show strictures but should not be performed in the acute phase due to high risk of bowel perforation.

Next steps in management

If NEC is clinically suspected, broad-spectrum antibiotic coverage, bowel rest, and imaging surveillance are instituted. Initial imaging studies usually consist of a supine and possibly also a cross-table lateral radiograph of the abdomen. This is followed by close interval follow-up at 8- to 12-hour intervals.

Further reading

1. Buonomo C. The radiology of necrotizing enterocolitis. Radiol Clin North Am. 1999 Nov;37(6):1187–1198, vii.
2. Epelman M, Daneman A, Navarro OM, et al. Necrotizing enterocolitis: review of state-of-the-art imaging findings with pathologic correlation. Radiographics. 2007 Mar–Apr;27(2):285–305.

History

▶ 15-year-old with abdominal pain and anorexia.

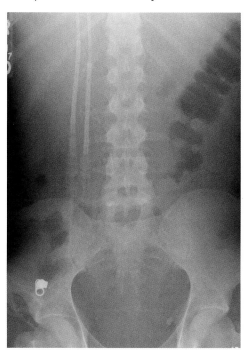

Case 37   Neutropenic Enterocolitis

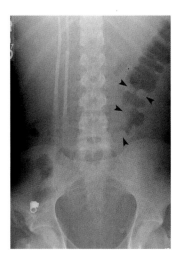

Findings

▶ The KUB shows thumbprinting of the haustra (arrowheads) and marked wall thickening of the right side of the transverse colon and no air in the ascending colon. The presence of the dual-lumen central venous catheter for chemotherapy suggests the diagnosis of neutropenic enterocolitis.

Differential diagnosis

The differential diagnosis for bowel wall thickening is quite broad. Considerations for predominantly right-sided involvement of the colon include yersinia, salmonella, tuberculosis, amebiasis, and neutropenic enterocolitis. Pseudomembranous colitis also occurs in patients on chemotherapy, though the rectosigmoid colon is usually involved. Ascites is common in pseudomembranous colitis but atypical in neutropenic enterocolitis.

Teaching points

▶ Neutropenic enterocolitis is a bacterial infection of the bowel most commonly seen in patients undergoing chemotherapy but also encountered in other immunocompromised patients, including those with organ transplantation, aplastic anemia, or HIV/AIDS.

▶ The condition was previously known as typhlitis, from the Greek word for cecum, *typhlon,* due to the fact that it most often affects the right colon. The left colon and the small bowel may also be involved.

▶ The imaging features are nonspecific and include mural thickening, pericolonic stranding and fluid, and pneumatosis. The process may be transmural and bowel perforation is a feared complication that should be sought on imaging. These features are well shown on CT, but limitation of radiation dose is desirable in oncology patients, who will undergo multiple follow-up exams. Ultrasound can also demonstrate these findings and can be performed at the bedside. Contrast enema is contraindicated.

▶ The mortality of neutropenic enterocolitis is about 20%, which is much lower than prior to the advent of early presumptive diagnosis and institution of supportive treatment.

Next steps in management

Early initiation of supportive treatment, including bowel rest and parenteral nutrition with broad-spectrum antibiotic coverage, often prevents complications requiring surgical intervention.

Further reading

1. Cronin CG, O'Connor M, Lohan DG, et al. Imaging of the gastrointestinal complications of systemic chemotherapy. Clin Radiol. 2009 Jul;64(7):724–733.
2. Dietrich CF. Significance of abdominal ultrasound in inflammatory bowel disease. Dig Dis. 2009;27(4):482–493.

History

► 5-month-old with abdominal pain.

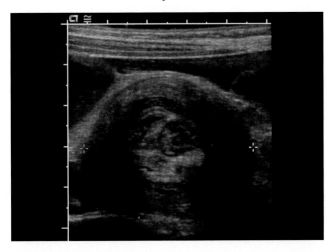

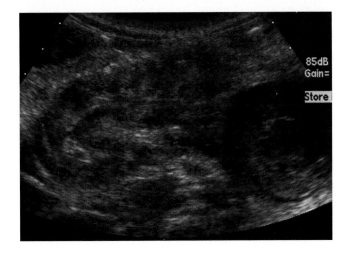

Case 38   Intussusception due to Duplication Cyst

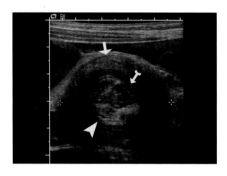 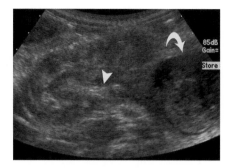

Findings

▶ On the transverse view (left), a round mass with the multilayered appearance of the wall of the intussuscepiens at the periphery (arrow) and of the intussusceptum (tailed arrow) surrounded by its echogenic mesenteric fat (arrowhead) in the center ("doughnut" sign).

▶ On the longitudinal view, the mass appears oblong with central echogenic mesenteric fat (arrowhead) ("pseudokidney" sign). The lead point, a duplication cyst containing debris, is also shown (curved arrow).

Differential diagnosis

The true finding of bowel within bowel is specific for intussusception, but bowel wall thickening, the normal psoas muscle in the transverse plane, or an intraluminal lipoma may produce an appearance similar to the doughnut sign.

Teaching points

▶ Intussusception is usually associated with viral gastroenteritis in children between 5 to 6 months and 3.5 years of age. Mesenteric adenopathy likely serves as the lead point. Patients outside this age range usually have a pathologic lead point, such as an inverted Meckel diverticulum (younger infants) or Burkitt lymphoma (older children). Other lead points include polyps (e.g., in Peutz-Jegher syndrome), enteric duplication cysts, inverted appendix, and intramural hematomas in Henoch-Schönlein purpura.

▶ Radiologic work-up begins with KUB and left lateral decubitus radiographs. If there is incomplete filling of the cecum with air, or if the exam is normal but clinical suspicion is very high, ultrasound is helpful in diagnosing or excluding intussusception, so that air or contrast enema can be reserved for treatment.

▶ On graded-compression ultrasound, findings associated with viral gastroenteritis, mesenteric adenopathy, and fluid-filled, hyperperistaltic bowel will also be seen. If the entire colon is examined in two planes with graded-compression technique and no uncompressible mass is found, colonic intussusception can be excluded.

Next steps in management

In the absence of contraindications (free air, peritoneal signs, or symptom duration greater than 24 hours), the intussusception may be reduced by contrast enema.

Further reading

1. Applegate KE. Intussusception in children: imaging choices. Semin Roentgenol. 2008 Jan;43(1):15.
2. Vasavada P. Ultrasound evaluation of acute abdominal emergencies. Radiol Clin North Am. 2004 Mar;42(2):445.

History

▶ 5-year-old girl with abdominal pain and skin rash on legs and buttocks.

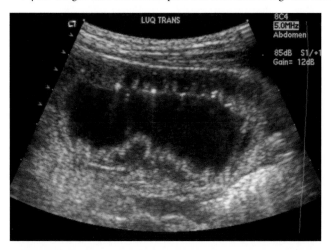

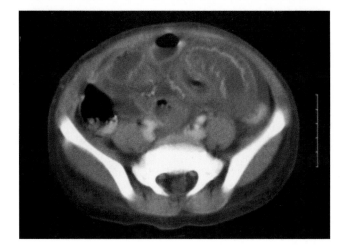

Case 39 Henoch-Schönlein Purpura

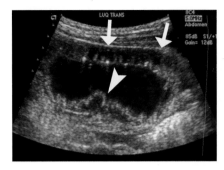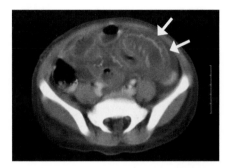

Findings

► Longitudinal ultrasound view of the small bowel (left) shows thickening of the bowel wall (arrows) and a focal area of thickening that may represent an intramural hemorrhage (arrowhead).
► CT image with IV contrast shows bowel wall thickening (arrows) with edema of the wall.

Differential diagnosis

Thickening of the bowel wall is a very abnormal but nonspecific finding. The differential includes infection (e.g., salmonella or yersinia), inflammation (e.g., Crohn disease, neutropenic enterocolitis, hemolytic uremic syndrome, or Henoch-Schönlein purpura), ischemia, or tumor (lymphoma). The lower-extremity skin rash and intramural hematoma in this case suggest the diagnosis of Henoch-Schönlein purpura.

Teaching points

► Henoch-Schönlein purpura is an idiopathic anaphylactoid reaction with vasculitis that may affect many organ systems. Patients may present with abdominal pain, arthritis, nephritis, or acute scrotum.
► The characteristic purpuric skin rash affects the lower extremities and buttocks more than the upper extremities and trunk. The rash suggests the diagnosis but often the abdominal pain precedes the development of the rash by several days.
► The jejunum is the most commonly affected part of the bowel. Intramural hematomas are frequent and may serve as the lead point for enteroenteric (small bowel–small bowel) intussusceptions. Unlike ileocolic intussusceptions, enteroenteric intussusceptions are usually self-limited.
► Imaging findings include small bowel wall thickening, focal areas of dilation alternating with areas of narrowing, submucosal masses, and enteroenteric intussusception.

Next steps in management

Management is supportive. Ultrasound is useful for following enteroenteric intussusceptions.

Further reading

1. Aideyan UO, Smith WL. Inflammatory bowel disease in children. Radiol Clin North Am. 1996 Jul;34(4):885–902.
2. Connolly B, O'Halpin D. Sonographic evaluation of the abdomen in Henoch-Schonlein purpura. Clin Radiol. 1994 May;49(5):320–323.

History

► Newborn boy with visible abnormality. Second image at age 4 months.

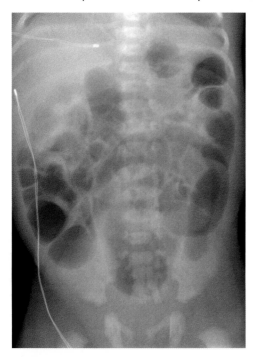

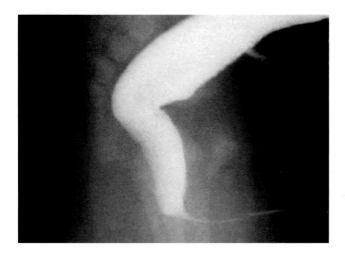

Case 40 Anorectal Malformation/VACTERL

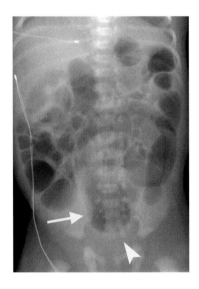

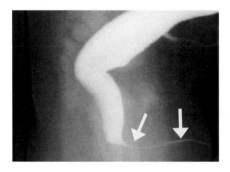

Findings

▸ KUB (left) shows multiple loops of dilated tubular bowel consistent with distal obstruction. The rectum (arrow) is also distended but does not extend to the symphysis pubis. Note also the presence of a sacral anomaly (arrowhead).

▸ Contrast opacification of the distal fistula after initial diverting colostomy (right) shows that the rectum connects to the urethra (arrows) rather than the perineum.

Differential diagnosis

Other causes of distal bowel obstruction in the newborn should be considered. Anorectal malformation is clinically diagnosed but is suggested on KUB by the presence of a dilated rectum.

Teaching points

▸ Anorectal malformation (imperforate anus) is due to lack of complete descent of the hindgut to the perineum and abnormal separation of the hindgut from the genitourinary (GU) tract.

▸ These malformations are designated as either high or low, depending on the degree of descent of the hindgut.
  ▪ Low malformations have a fistulous opening on the perineum, which represents the termination of the hindgut.
  ▪ High malformations have a fistula to a GU tract structure immediately anterior to the hindgut. For boys, this is the bladder or urethra. For girls, it is the vagina or vestibule. High malformations have a worse prognosis for rectal continence, because it is the descent of the hindgut in the pelvis that induces the development of the levator sling.

▸ Anorectal malformation is associated with VACTERL, GU anomalies, lumbosacral spine anomalies, and tethered cord. The Currarino triad comprises anorectal malformation, presacral mass, and sacral anomaly.

Next steps in management

Other findings of VACTERL should be sought on radiographs. Renal ultrasound and MR of the spine are helpful. Initial treatment is a diverting colostomy shortly after birth, followed by definitive repair at 6 months of age. Low lesions are approached from the perineum, while high lesions require an abdominal and perineal approach.

Further reading

1. Buonomo C. Neonatal gastrointestinal emergencies. Radiol Clin North Am. 1997;35:845–864.
2. Masi P, Miele E, Staiano A. Pediatric anorectal disorders. Gastroenterol Clin North Am. 2008;37:709–730.

History

▸ 2-day-old with distention.

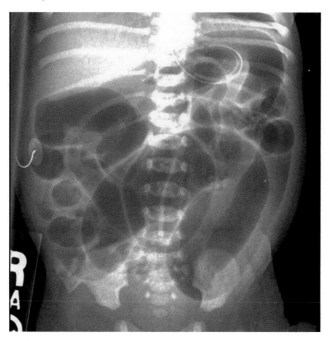

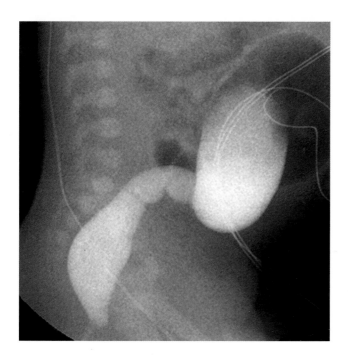

Case 41   Hirschsprung Disease

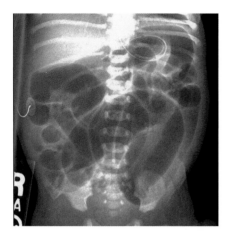 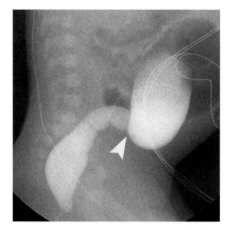

Findings

▶ KUB (left) shows multiple dilated tubular loops of bowel and absence of rectal air.
▶ Contrast enema shows a transition zone in the sigmoid colon (arrowhead) and rectosigmoid ratio of less than 1.

Differential diagnosis

In the newborn, the differential diagnosis of distal bowel obstruction also includes congenital atresias and functional immaturity. For older infants, the main differential consideration is functional constipation.

Teaching points

▶ Hirschsprung disease is caused by an absence of ganglion cells in the muscle wall of the distal colon, preventing relaxation of the affected segment.
▶ As a result of this functional obstruction, the normal proximal bowel dilates over time, creating a funnel-shaped transition zone, which may not be discernable at birth. A normal contrast enema in the neonatal period should not dissuade one from performing another enema later if constipation persists.
▶ In most patients, the affected bowel is the rectosigmoid colon (short segment) but longer portions of the colon can be affected (intermediate/long segment). Total colonic Hirschsprung disease is inherited and rare.
▶ Most but not all patients present with failure to pass meconium within the first 24 hours of life. Males are more commonly affected.
▶ When performing a contrast enema, never inflate a balloon in the rectum of a child, as the balloon could rupture the aganglionic segment. Start with a lateral view of the rectosigmoid colon, which best shows the transition zone. Stop filling once the transition zone is demonstrated.
▶ Barium is inert and may be used for the older infant. For newborns, bowel perforation may be present without free air, so dilute water-soluble contrast is preferred.
▶ Untreated Hirschsprung patients can develop necrotizing enterocolitis (NEC). Do not perform an enema if the infant has signs or symptoms of NEC.

Next steps in management

Treatment is surgical resection of the continuous aganglionic segment and anal pull-through.

Further reading

1. Buonomo C. Neonatal gastrointestinal emergencies. Radiol Clin North Am 1997;35:845–864.
2. Cohen MD. Choosing contrast media for the evaluation of the gastrointestinal tract of neonates and infants. Radiology 1987;162:447–456.

History

▶ 2-day-old with abdominal distention.

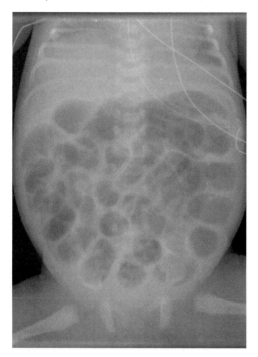

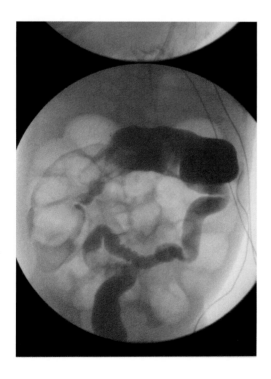

Case 42 Functional Immaturity of the Colon

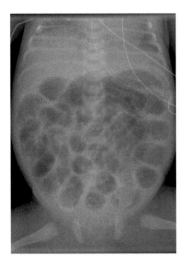 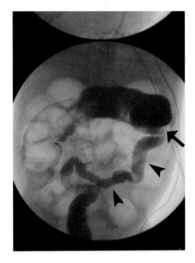

Findings

- ▸ KUB (left) shows many distended, tubular loops of bowel consistent with distal obstruction.
- ▸ Contrast enema (right) demonstrates small caliber of the left colon (arrowheads) but normal rectosigmoid ratio, and an abrupt transition at the splenic flexure (arrow). The patient passed a meconium plug at the end of the procedure.

Differential diagnosis

See Case 26.

Teaching points

- ▸ Nomenclature—This condition was previously known as *meconium plug syndrome*, but now it is recognized that not all patients with functional immaturity of the colon have meconium plugs, and not all patients with meconium plugs have functional immaturity. Other causes of meconium plug include Hirschsprung disease and cystic fibrosis. Thus, meconium plug is a symptom, not a syndrome. Functional immaturity is also known as *neonatal small left colon syndrome*, a name that describes its appearance on contrast enema. The name *functional immaturity of the colon* reflects its clinical course.
- ▸ Functional immaturity occurs in infants of diabetic mothers or whose mothers were treated with magnesium sulfate. Patients experience clinical improvement after the enema and may pass a meconium plug following the enema. Symptoms resolve completely within days to weeks.
- ▸ On the contrast enema the left colon and rectosigmoid colon are abnormally small in caliber and there is an abrupt transition from normal to abnormal caliber at the splenic flexure.
- ▸ Versus Hirschsprung disease—In functional immaturity, the transition zone is abrupt (vs. gradual and funnel-shaped in Hirschsprung disease) and always located at the splenic flexure (vs. rectosigmoid colon), and the left colon is small (vs. normal caliber with dilated proximal colon).

Next steps in management

Treatment is medical. The enema is therapeutic.

Further reading

1. Buonomo C. Neonatal gastrointestinal emergencies. Radiologic Clinics of North America 1997;35: 845–864.
2. Ellis H, Kumar R, Kostyrka B. Neonatal small left colon syndrome in the offspring of diabetic mothers—an analysis of 105 children. J Pediatr Surg. 2009 Dec;44(12):2343–2346.

History

▶ 12-year-old girl with fever and right lower quadrant pain.

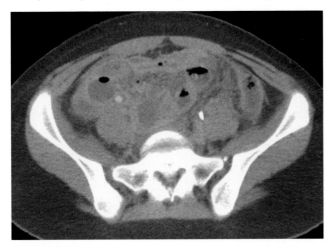

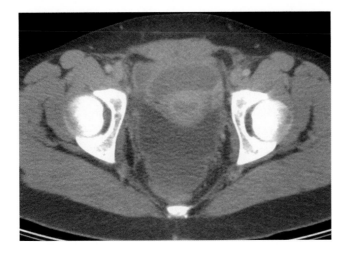

Case 43 Appendiceal Abscess with Appendicolith

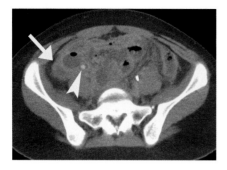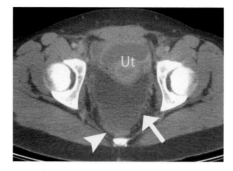

Findings

▶ Image from a CT scan after IV contrast (left) shows inflammation and fluid in the right paracolic gutter (arrow) and a round calcification representing an appendicolith (arrowhead).

▶ Lower image (right) reveals a fluid collection with enhancing margin (arrow) in the space between the uterus (Ut) and the rectum (arrowhead).

Differential diagnosis

Pelvic abscess in an adolescent girl may be due to perforated appendicitis, Crohn disease, or pelvic inflammatory disease (PID). An appendicolith indicates appendicitis.

Teaching points

▶ Children are more likely to have a perforated appendix at surgery and children have a higher negative laparotomy rate compared to adults.

▶ Graded-compression ultrasound is preferred for the evaluation of young children. The obstructed appendix appears as a blind-ending, uncompressible loop of bowel with multilayered wall (gut signature).

▶ The size criterion for an enlarged appendix is the same in children as it is in adults—greater than 6 mm in diameter as measured from one outer wall to the opposite outer wall.

▶ CT examination for appendicitis has high sensitivity and specificity in children but the disadvantage of radiation exposure. Oral and IV contrast should be used in imaging young children for appendicitis because children lack body fat and have less internal contrast on CT. Rectal contrast is well tolerated by children and can be administered more rapidly than oral contrast.

▶ Potential pitfalls on imaging:

  ▪ Tip appendicitis—one must visualize the entire length of the appendix in order to call it normal
  ▪ Ruptured appendicitis—once ruptured, the inflamed appendix is usually no longer dilated

Next steps in management

The treatment for an unruptured appendicitis is laparoscopic appendectomy. For ruptured appendicitis, the treatment is percutaneous or transrectal drainage of the abscess.

Further reading

1. Rosendahl K, Aukland SM, Fosse K. Imaging strategies in children with suspected appendicitis. Eur Radiol. 2004 Mar;12 Suppl 4:L138–L145.
2. Sivit CJ, Siegel MJ, Applegate KE, Newman KD. When appendicitis suspected in children. Radiographics. 2001 Jan–Feb;21(1):247–262.

History

▶ Newborn premature infant.

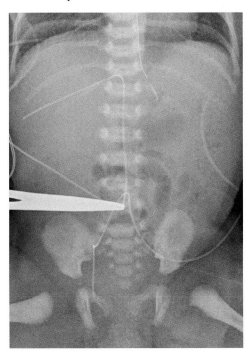

Case 44 Misplaced Umbilical Artery and Vein Catheters

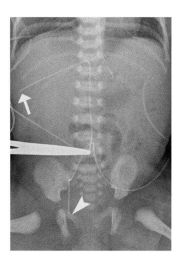

Findings

▶ AP radiograph of the abdomen demonstrates an umbilical venous catheter coursing through the umbilical vein recess and ductus venosus into the left then right portal vein, where it terminates (arrow). An umbilical arterial catheter is coursing caudally to the internal iliac artery and then into the distal common iliac artery to terminate in the common femoral artery (arrowhead).

Differential diagnosis

None.

Teaching points

▶ The normal course of the umbilical venous catheter (UVC) is through the umbilical vein to the umbilical vein recess (also called umbilical sinus) to the ductus venosus to the inferior vena cava at the hepatic venous confluence just below the inferior cavoatrial junction. The desired position of the catheter tip is at the inferior cavoatrial junction or just within the right atrium. The umbilical vein recess is contiguous with the left portal vein, so malposition within the portal venous system may occur, possibly leading to portal vein thrombosis or hepatic laceration or abscess formation.

▶ On the lateral view, the expected course of the UVC is superficial in the umbilical vein, then turning posterior at the inferior liver margin as it enters the umbilical vein recess, forming an upward-bowing convexity. The catheter then forms an upward concavity as it enters the sinus venosus toward the intrahepatic inferior vena cava.

▶ The normal course of the umbilical arterial catheter is caudad through one of the umbilical arteries to the internal iliac artery, then cephalad through the common iliac artery to the aorta. The preferred position is in the thoracic aorta, usually between the level of T6 and T10. This location is associated with the least risk of thromboembolic events involving the mesenteric, renal, and lower extremity circulation.

Next steps in management

The catheters must be withdrawn and repositioned.

Further reading

1. Oestreich AE. Umbilical vein catheterization—appropriate and inappropriate placement. Pediatr Radiol. 2010 Dec;40(12):1941–1949.
2. Narla LD, Hom M, Lofland GK, Moskowitz WB. Evaluation of umbilical catheter and tube placement in premature infants. Radiographics. 1991 Sep;11(5):849–863.

History

► 2-week-old with emesis.

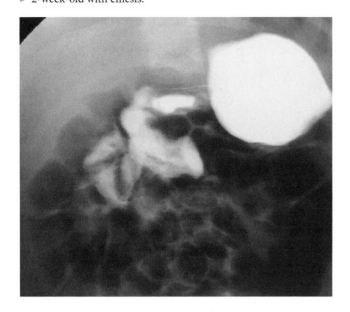

Case 45 Malrotation

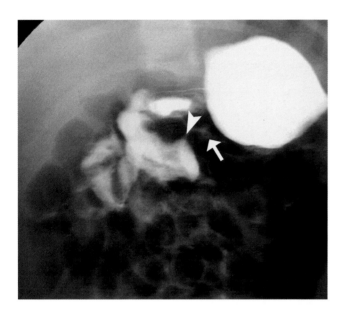

Findings

▶ AP image from an upper GI series shows that the duodenal–jejunal junction (DJJ) (arrowhead) is low and located to the right of the left pedicle of L1 (arrow).

Differential diagnosis

The imaging differential diagnosis for emesis in a young infant depends on the character of the emesis. Bilious emesis suggests an obstruction distal to the ampulla of Vater. The diagnosis that must be excluded is midgut volvulus.

Teaching points

▶ Malrotation is a congenital anomaly of bowel development that predisposes the patient to midgut volvulus.

▶ The best imaging study for suspected malrotation/midgut volvulus is the upper GI series. Demonstration of the normal DJJ has a very high negative predictive value. The normal position of the DJJ is on or to the left of the left pedicle of usually L1. The top of the DJJ should rise at least as high as the bottom of the duodenal bulb. The location of the DJJ should be demonstrated on all pediatric upper GI series.

▶ Technical considerations

■ The patient must be perfectly positioned in the AP projection when evaluating the position of the DJJ as rotation can cause spurious results.

■ The stomach distended with air can displace the DJJ slightly downward and rightward.

▶ If the location of the DJJ is normal, the patient does not have malrotation; however, sometimes the location of the DJJ is equivocal. The exam can be repeated after the stomach is emptied of air. It may be helpful to complete a small bowel follow-through looking for high cecum or jejunum in the right upper quadrant or to perform an ultrasound to look for superior mesenteric artery/vein inversion indicating malrotation.

Next steps in management

The treatment for malrotation is the Ladd procedure.

Further reading

1. Strouse PJ. Disorders of intestinal rotation and fixation ("malrotation"). Pediatr Radiol 2004;34:837–851.
2. Applegate KE, Anderson JM, Klatte EC. Intestinal malrotation in children: a problem-solving approach to the upper gastrointestinal series. Radiographics 200;26(5):1485–1500.

History

▶ 4-year-old boy with abdominal pain, fever, nausea, and vomiting.

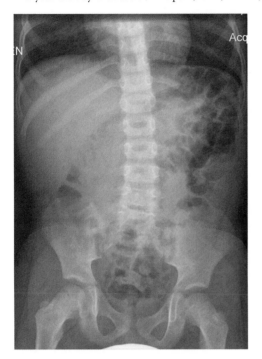

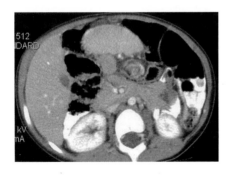
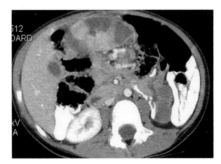

Case 46 Wandering Spleen with Volvulus and Infarction

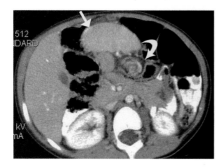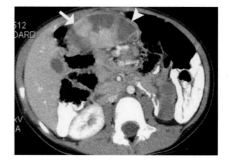

Findings

- ► KUB (see opposite page) shows absence of the expected spleen shadow in the left upper quadrant.
- ► Axial CT images show the low midline mass shaped like the spleen (arrow) with foci of decreased enhancement (arrowhead) with preservation of enhancement of the capsule. The whirl sign of twisted vessels of the splenic hilum is noted (curved arrow).

Differential diagnosis

Absence of the spleen shadow could also be due to splenic infarction due to sickle cell anemia or due to polysplenia with multiple small spleens. Other findings suggesting sickle cell disease could include enlarged heart and avascular necrosis of the femoral heads. Other findings suggesting polysplenia could include situs anomalies.

Teaching points

- ► Wandering spleen is a rare condition in which the spleen is found in the abdomen due to a defect in its ligamentous fixation, which may be congenital. About one third of cases are diagnosed in children.
- ► Wandering spleen may be found incidentally or may cause severe abdominal pain due to torsion around its vascular pedicle. Persistent torsion can lead to infarction and represents a surgical emergency.
- ► Unexplained absence of the spleen from its normal location is a very helpful finding. The untorsed ectopic spleen resembles a normal spleen but the infarcted spleen is enlarged and hypoattenuating to liver, and is not as easily recognized as the spleen. A rim of enhancement of the splenic capsule due to collateral circulation is common. The whirl sign is specific for torsion.
- ► The pancreatic tail may also be involved in the torsion is some cases.

Next steps in management

Untorsed wandering spleens are treated with splenopexy, but if the spleen is infarcted, splenectomy is required.

Further reading

1. Ben Ely A, Zissin R, Copel L, et al. The wandering spleen: CT findings and possible pitfalls in diagnosis. Clin Radiol. 2006 Nov;61(11):954–958.
2. Bakir B, Poyanli A, Yekeler E, Acunas G. Acute torsion of a wandering spleen: imaging findings. Abdom Imaging. 2004 Nov–Dec;29(6):707–709.

Part 3   Genitourinary System

History

▶ 3-year-old with UTI.

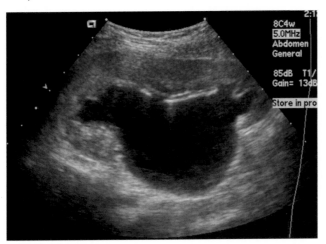

Case 47 Ureteropelvic Junction Obstruction

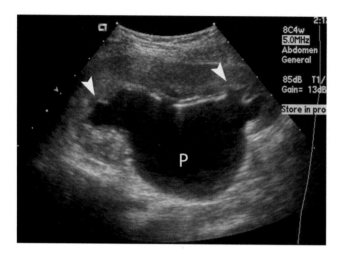

Findings

▸ Longitudinal ultrasound image shows a dilated, bulbous renal pelvis (P) and blunted calyces (arrowheads), but no dilated ureter. Normal-appearing renal parenchyma is noted.

Differential diagnosis

Cystic masses originating from the kidney include ureteropelvic junction (UPJ) obstruction, multicystic dysplastic kidney (MCDK), and multilocular cystic renal tumor. The finding of renal parenchyma around the cyst excludes MCDK. The continuity of the cyst with the dilated intrarenal collecting system indicates the diagnosis of obstruction. The absence of a dilated ureter localizes the obstruction to the UPJ.

Teaching points

▸ UPJ obstruction is the most common cause of upper tract obstruction in children. In the past, patients presented with symptoms of fever, flank pain, mass, hematuria, or UPJ avulsion following trauma. Now, most patients are diagnosed prenatally.
▸ Lasix renography shows an obstructive time–activity curve.
▸ Associations: abnormality of contralateral kidney (most commonly UPJ obstruction) and renal dysplasia
▸ UPJ obstruction may be due to intrinsic or extrinsic causes. Extrinsic UPJ obstruction is due to crossing vessels. These patients have lesser degrees of obstruction with intermittent symptoms and findings during diuretic periods (Dietl's crisis). Half of patients who are diagnosed with symptoms rather than prenatally have crossing vessels.

Next steps in management

Mild to moderate cases are followed and treated if they worsen or become symptomatic. Severe obstruction in young children is treated with dismembered pyeloplasty. Adolescents and adults diagnosed with UPJ obstruction are candidates for a ureteroscopic procedure called endopyelotomy. Patients with the extrinsic form of UPJ obstruction are not candidates for endopyelotomy due to the high risk of hemorrhagic complications. For this reason, patients who present with symptoms undergo preoperative CT or MR angiography to evaluate for the presence of a crossing vessel.

Further reading

1. Rooks VJ, Lebowitz RL. Extrinsic ureteropelvic junction obstruction from a crossing vessel: demography and imaging. Pediatr Radiol. 2001 Feb;31(2):120–124.
2. Calder AD, Hiorns MP, Abhyankar A, et al. Contrast-enhanced magnetic resonance angiography for the detection of crossing renal vessels in children with symptomatic UPJ obstruction. Pediatr Radiol. 2007 Apr;37(4):356–361.

History

▶ Newborn with prenatal diagnosis of abnormal right kidney.

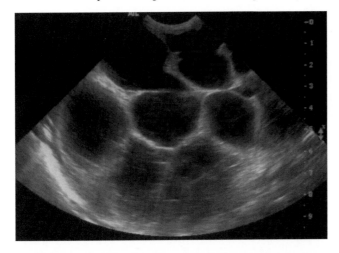

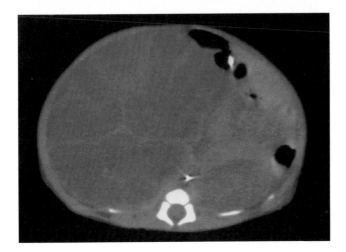

Case 48 Multicystic Dysplastic Kidney (MCDK)

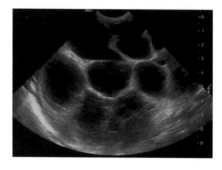 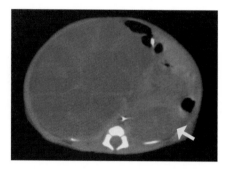

Findings

- ▶ Longitudinal ultrasound image (left) of the right abdomen shows a multilocular cyst and no normal renal parenchyma.
- ▶ Axial unenhanced CT image (right) demonstrates the multilocular cyst and left kidney (arrow).

Differential diagnosis

Failure to find a displaced normal right kidney suggests a renal origin with a differential of ureteropelvic junction (UPJ) obstruction and multicystic dysplastic kidney (MCDK). Multilocular appearance and absence of surrounding normal renal parenchyma indicates a diagnosis of MCDK. In an older infant the differential would include multilocular cystic renal tumor, which is distinguished by the presence of surrounding renal parenchyma.

Teaching points

- ▶ MCDK is the most common cause of renal mass found in the first week of life.
- ▶ In utero obstruction to urine flow results in renal dysplasia, and MCDK is the extreme end of the spectrum of UPJ obstruction involving the infundibulopelvis, resulting in a mass of noncommunicating macrocysts with no normal renal parenchyma.
- ▶ The condition is rarely bilateral (incompatible with life). There is a risk of abnormality of the opposite kidney—UPJ obstruction or vesicoureteral reflux (VUR) (25%). The opposite kidney is the solitary functioning kidney and it should be screened for VUR.
- ▶ In the classic form, the noncommunicating cysts are of varying sizes with no large central cyst and the mass is usually nonreniform. In the hydronephrotic form (10%) there may be a large central cyst and the cysts may communicate. This form may be impossible to differentiate from severe UPJ obstruction with compressed parenchyma.
- ▶ The natural history is to resolve in most cases.

Next steps in management

The patient should undergo annual follow-up ultrasound until resolution. Those that fail to resolve or get larger are resected due to the small risk of malignant transformation.

Further reading

1. Thomsen HS, Levine E, Meilstrup JW, et al. Renal cystic diseases. Eur Radiol. 1997;7(8):1267–1275.
2. Wootton-Gorges SL, Thomas KB, Harned RK, et al. Giant cystic abdominal masses in children. Pediatr Radiol. 2005 Dec;35(12):1277–1288.

History

▶ Newborn boy with abnormal prenatal ultrasound.

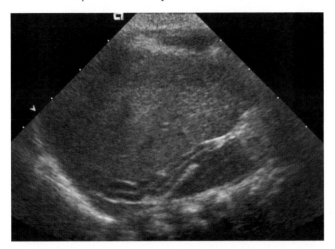

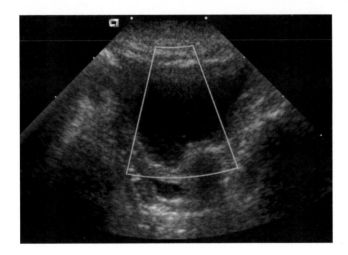

Case 49 Right Renal Agenesis with Seminal Vesicle Cyst

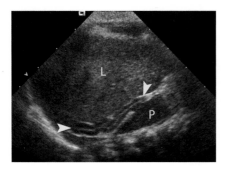 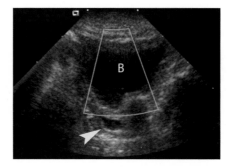

Findings

▶ Longitudinal ultrasound image of the right renal fossa shows an elongated structure with echogenic linear core surrounded by hypoechoic rim (arrowheads) behind the liver (L) and anterior to the psoas muscle (P).

▶ Transverse ultrasound image reveals a cystic structure (arrowhead) posterior to the bladder (B) on the right, which represents a seminal vesicle cyst.

Differential diagnosis

The elongated appearance of the adrenal gland mimics the appearance of a small kidney. Absence of the kidney from the renal fossa could also be due to ectopia of the kidney. In an older child or adult, absence of the kidney could be due to resolution of a multicystic dysplastic kidney.

Teaching points

▶ If only one kidney is identified in the orthotopic location and it is enlarged, then it is the only functioning kidney. On the other hand, compensatory hypertrophy of the solitary functioning kidney may not develop until after age 6 to 12 months.

▶ In young infants, the adrenal gland is relatively easy to see on ultrasound. In the presence of the adjacent kidney, the adrenal gland assumes a Y- or V-shaped configuration. Without an adjacent kidney, the adrenal gland is straight and elongated in appearance. The adrenal medulla is echogenic and the cortex is hypoechoic, so the adrenal gland may be mistaken for a small kidney.

▶ Associated genital anomalies are seen in 25%:
  ▪ Mullerian fusion anomalies for girls
  ▪ Seminal vesicle cysts for boys ipsilateral to the agenesis

Next steps in management

If there is compensatory hypertrophy of the observed kidney, there is no need to search for another. Otherwise, ultrasound of pelvis is indicated, followed by renal cortical scintigraphy, if necessary. If the observed kidney is a solitary kidney, vesicoureteral reflux should be excluded in a young child.

Further reading

1. Daneman A, Alton DJ. Radiographic manifestations of renal anomalies. Radiol Clin North Am. 1991;29:351–363.
2. Mercado-Deane MG, Beeson JE, John SD. US of renal insufficiency in neonates. Radiographics. 2002 Nov–Dec;22(6): 1429–1438.

History

▶ 3-year-old girl with UTI.

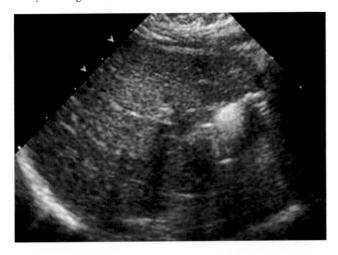

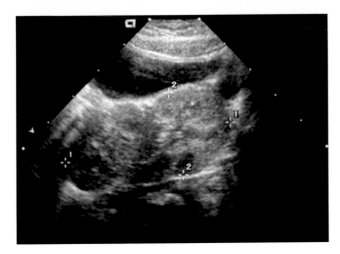

Case 50   Renal Ectopia

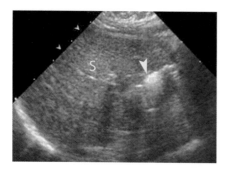 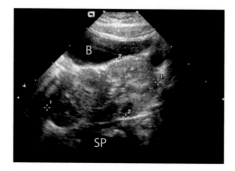

Findings

▶ Longitudinal US image (left) of the left renal fossa shows only shadowing bowel gas (arrowhead) behind the spleen (S).

▶ Longitudinal US image of the pelvis (right) shows a small, slightly dysmorphic kidney (calipers) posterior to the bladder (B) and anterior to the spine (SP).

Differential diagnosis

Ectopic kidneys are often small and slightly dysmorphic with an eccentric, superficial, or absent renal sinus. Since it is the location, reniform shape, and central fat that allow us to identify the kidney on imaging studies, the ectopic kidney may be mistaken for a pelvic mass such as organ of Zückerkandl neuroblastoma or ovarian tumor.

Teaching points

▶ Congenital renal anomalies include ectopia, fusion, and malrotation (abnormal position of the renal sinus), which often occur together.

▶ Renal ectopia may be simple (orthotopic side) or crossed (both kidneys on the same side of the body). Crossed ectopic kidneys are almost always fused to the other kidney (crossed fused ectopia). The lower portion is always the ectopic kidney. The ureter of the ectopic kidney crosses to the other side to insert orthotopically into the bladder.

▶ The most common site of the ectopic kidney is the pelvis. The most common form of fusion is the horseshoe kidney. In young children, the parenchymal isthmus of the horseshoe kidney may be visible on ultrasound in the midline. Cake or lump kidney results from complete failure of the metanephros to separate into two parts and to rise out of the pelvis.

▶ Ectopic kidneys are at slightly increased risk for trauma, stone formation, infection, renovascular hypertension, and tumors.

Next steps in management

Ectopic kidneys are generally asymptomatic and require no treatment. The prenatal finding of a renal anomaly should prompt a search for anomalies of other organ systems or evidence of syndromes associated with renal anomalies, such as VACTERL association or Turner syndrome.

Further reading

1. de Bruyn R, Marks SD. Postnatal investigation of fetal renal disease. Semin Fetal Neonatal Med. 2008 June;13(3):133–141.
2. Cohen HL, Kravets F, Zucconi W, et al. Congenital abnormalities of the genitourinary system. Semin Roentgenol. 2004 Apr:39(2):282–303.

History

► Newborn 26-week premature boy.

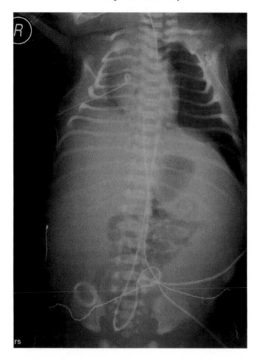

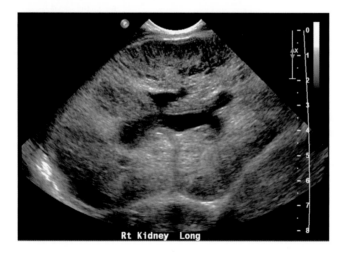

Case 51 Autosomal Recessive Polycystic Kidney Disease (ARPKD)

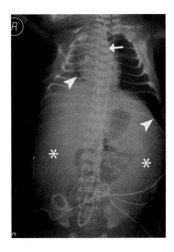 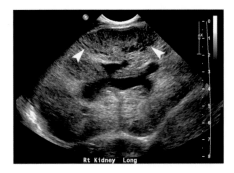

Findings

▸ Supine AP radiograph (left) shows small bell-shaped thorax, bilateral pneumothoraces (arrowheads), bilateral chest tubes, and endotracheal tube (arrow). Bilateral flank masses (*) push bowel gas centrally.

▸ Longitudinal renal US shows increased echogenicity. Dilated tubules can be resolved (arrowheads).

Differential diagnosis

For the plain radiographic appearance, the differential includes bilateral multicystic dysplastic kidneys and Eagle Barrett syndrome.

Teaching points

▸ ARPKD is a disease of the kidneys and the liver. The kidneys are involved with ectasia of the collecting tubules and the liver with congenital hepatic fibrosis and biliary duct ectasia. The degrees of renal and hepatic involvement are inversely proportional and determine a spectrum of clinical presentation. Patients with a lot of renal disease present in the perinatal period with oligohydramnios and pulmonary hypoplasia, while patients with predominantly liver disease present in childhood with symptoms of portal hypertension.

▸ In infants, the kidneys are enlarged and diffusely echogenic on ultrasound. The "cysts" are actually dilated collecting tubules in the renal medullae. These tubules are oriented radially. These dilated tubules are only 1 to 2 mm in diameter, and the kidneys are echogenic because the multiple cyst walls reflect the sound wave back to the transducer. Modern ultrasound equipment allows resolution of these small tubular cysts. A dark halo of compressed cortex is seen in half of patients.

▸ Patients who present later with liver disease have imaging findings of portal hypertension. They may have dilated biliary ducts, occasionally so large that they engulf the portal venous radical (target sign).

Next steps in management

Management and prognosis depend on clinical presentation. Those with severe renal involvement die in the perinatal period from pulmonary hypoplasia. Those who present with liver disease are medically managed, though they may later require liver transplant.

Further reading

1. Lonergan GJ, Rice RR, Suarez ES. Autosomal recessive polycystic kidney disease: radiologic-pathologic correlation. Radiographics. 2000 May–Jun;20(3):837–855.
2. Turkbey B, Ocak I, Daryanani K, et al. Autosomal recessive polycystic kidney disease and congenital hepatic fibrosis (ARPKD/CHF). Pediatr Radiol. 2009 Feb;39(2):100–111.

History

► 4-year-old girl with fever.

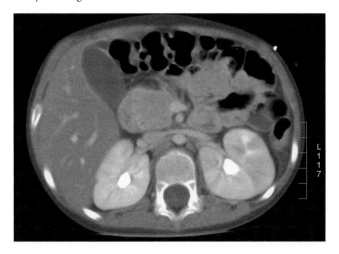

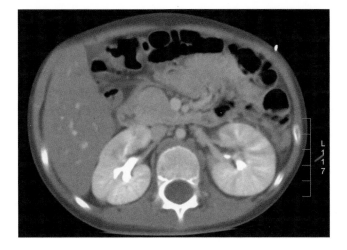

Case 52 Acute Multifocal Pyelonephritis

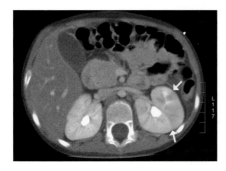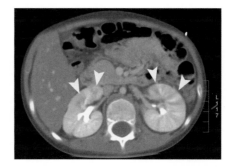

Findings

▶ Axial enhanced image (left) reveals a wedge-shaped focus of decreased enhancement between the two arrows.

▶ CT image (right) shows a streaky, inhomogeneous enhancement pattern bilaterally (arrowheads).

Differential diagnosis

The heterogeneous enhancement pattern in a febrile patient is specific for pyelonephritis.

Teaching points

▶ In children outside the neonatal period, pyelonephritis is generally an ascending infection. Although the relationship between vesicoureteral reflux (VUR) and renal scarring is controversial, the current rationale for screening and treating patients for VUR is the belief that three conditions are required for children to develop renal scarring: UTI, VUR, and intrarenal reflux. If one of these is absent, scarring will not occur.

▶ Intrarenal reflux occurs in compound papillae that are found at the poles, upper more than lower, and pyelonephritis is most often found at the poles. Other factors also predispose to scarring, including bladder dysfunction and urinary tract malformation.

▶ Infants usually present with fever. Older children have more specific findings. If the clinical picture is straightforward, no imaging is required. If the patient fails to improve with adequate therapy after 24 to 48 hours, then imaging is indicated to evaluate for abscess or pyonephrosis.

▶ Ultrasound is not as sensitive as CT, MRI, or renal cortical scintigraphy. On all modalities the abnormalities may be unifocal, multifocal, bilateral, or diffuse. The affected area is usually wedge-shaped and has decreased enhancement/perfusion compared to adjacent kidney. The involved area is enlarged due to edema and inflammatory infiltrate.

Next steps in management

Patients with simple pyelonephritis are treated with IV antibiotics. Those with complications are treated with drainage. Patients should undergo screening for reflux, which can be performed while hospitalized to prevent loss to follow-up.

Further reading

1. Orellana P, Baquedano P, Rangarajan V. Relationship between acute pyelonephritis, renal scarring and vesicoureteral reflux. Results of a coordinated research project. Pediatr Nephrol. 2004;19:1122–1126.
2. Smith EA. Pyelonephritis, renal scarring, and reflux nephropathy: a pediatric urologist's perspective. Pediatr Radiol. 2008 Jan;38 Suppl 1:S76–S82.

History

▶ 6-year-old girl with febrile UTI.

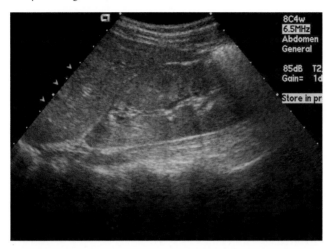

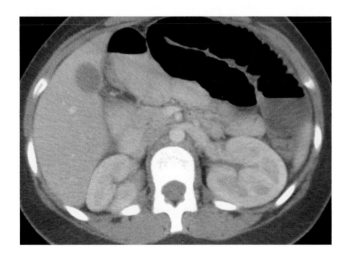

Case 53 Renal Scarring—Reflux Nephropathy

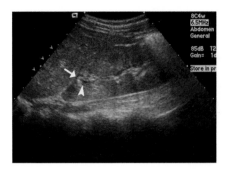 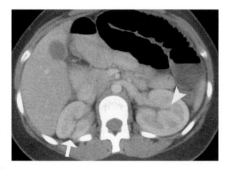

Findings

▶ Longitudinal ultrasound of the right kidney shows a parenchymal defect in the upper pole (arrow), so that the calyx (arrowhead) nearly touches the liver.

▶ Axial CT shows a tissue defect in the right posterior upper pole (arrow). The calyx extends to the surface of the kidney. Compare to the normal appearance of a calyx on the left (arrowhead), which is covered by the medullary pyramid and adjacent renal cortex.

Differential diagnosis

The full-thickness destruction of the parenchyma causes a defect over a calyx, which is specific for renal scarring. Fetal lobulation appears as an indentation between calyces.

Teaching points

▶ Reflux nephropathy (renal scarring or post-infectious nephropathy) is the sequela of pyelonephritis. Like pyelonephritis, the abnormality involves the full thickness of the parenchyma, is centered over the calyx, and is more common at the poles, upper more than lower. There is destruction of parenchyma with volume loss and replacement with fibrous scar. Without the adjacent papilla, the calyx loses its cup shape and becomes blunted.

▶ Ultrasound is less sensitive for scarring than CT, MRI, or renal cortical scintigraphy. With diffuse scarring, ultrasound may show only lack of growth or a small kidney for age. Evaluation of renal size and comparison to the other kidney, to old studies, or to an age-based nomogram is important in the US evaluation of children with UTI. The maximum tolerated size difference between the two kidneys is 5 mm for children.

Next steps in management

Renal scar is usually caused by ascending infection from vesicoureteral reflux. A voiding cystourethrogram is indicated if the diagnosis of reflux is not already established.

Further reading

1. Elder JS, Peters CA, Arant BS Jr, et al. Pediatric vesicoureteral reflux guidelines panel summary report of primary vesi-coureteral reflux in children. J Urol 1997;157:1846–1851.
2. Ricccabona M, Avnie FE, Blickman JG, et al. Imaging recommendations in paediatric uroradiology: minutes of the ESPR workgroup session on urinary tract infection, fetal hydronephrosis, urinary tract ultrasonography, and voiding cystoure-thrography, Barcelona, Spain, June 2007. Pediatr Radiol. 2008;38:138–145.

History

▶ 15-month-old boy with increasing abdominal girth.

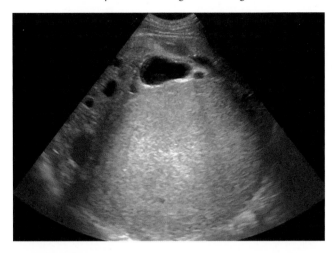

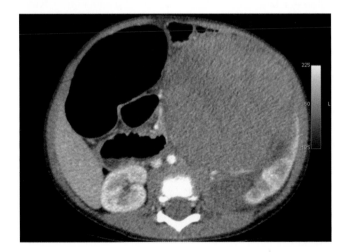

Case 54 Wilms' Tumor

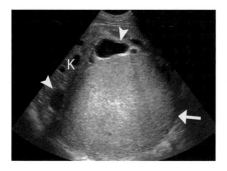 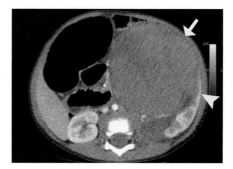

Findings

▶ Longitudinal ultrasound image (left) reveals a homogeneous mass (arrow) arising from the left kidney (K) and causing hydronephrosis (arrowheads).

▶ Axial enhanced CT image (right) shows the homogenous mass (arrow) and the claw sign (arrowhead).

Differential diagnosis

Wilms' is the most common renal tumor in this age group. The most important differential consideration is adrenal neuroblastoma. Other renal tumors include clear cell sarcoma of the kidney, rhabdoid tumor, multilocular cystic renal tumor, and renal cell carcinoma (RCC). Multilocular cystic renal tumor is cystic. The other tumors cannot be distinguished from Wilms' on the basis of imaging features, but RCC usually occurs in older children.

Teaching points

▶ Wilms' tumor, or nephroblastoma, is an embryonal tumor and the most common abdominal malignancy in children.

▶ The peak age of incidence is 3 to 4 years, which overlaps with the age of incidence of another common tumor that often arises in a similar location—neuroblastoma. Differentiating features are as follows:

  ▪ Renal claw sign in Wilms' versus renal displacement in neuroblastoma

  ▪ Calcification is common in neuroblastoma but uncommon in Wilms'.

  ▪ Neuroblastoma tends to encase vessels, while Wilms' tumor may invade veins.

  ▪ Neuroblastoma commonly crosses midline and may invade neural foramina, features that are rare in Wilms'.

  ▪ Wilms' tumor metastasizes to lung, while neuroblastoma spreads to liver and bone.

▶ On imaging, the appearance is variable. Wilms' enhances less than the adjacent kidney.

▶ Bilateral Wilms' (stage V disease) is virtually always associated with a syndrome and nephroblastomatosis.

Next steps in management

CT of the chest and MR or CT of the abdomen are helpful for staging prior to nephrectomy. Careful evaluation of the renal vein for invasion is required.

Further reading

1. Lowe LH, Isuani BH, Heller RM, et al. Pediatric renal masses: Wilms tumor and beyond. Radiographics. 2000 Nov–Dec;20(6):1585–1603.
2. Smets AM, de Kraker J. Malignant tumours of the kidney: imaging strategy. Pediatr Radiol. 2010 Jun;40(6):1010–1018.

History

▶ 10-month-old with abdominal mass.

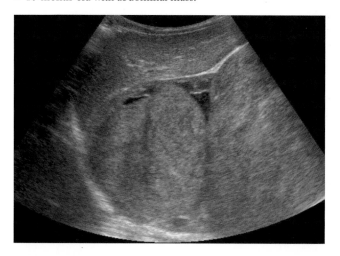

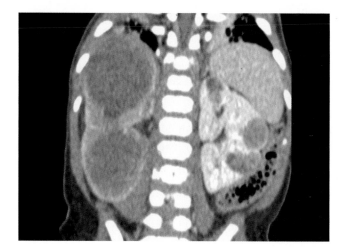

Case 55 Right Wilms' Tumor and Nephroblastomatosis

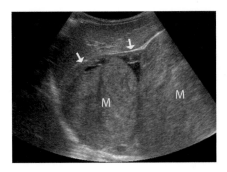
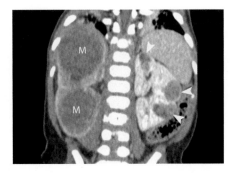

Findings

▶ Longitudinal ultrasound image (left) reveals a bilobed homogeneous mass (M) arising from the right kidney (arrows).
▶ Coronal reformatted CT image (right) shows the right mass (M) as well as several hypo-enhancing masses in the left kidney (arrowheads), some of which are triangular. The middle, round mass was also a Wilms' tumor.

Differential diagnosis

With masses in both kidneys, the differential diagnosis is narrowed to Wilms' tumor and nephrogenic rests.

Teaching points

▶ A nephrogenic rest is a persistent focus of metanephric blastema beyond 36 weeks gestation, and nephroblastomatosis is the condition of multiple or diffuse nephrogenic rests.
▶ Most nephrogenic rests will spontaneously mature into normal renal tissue, but occasionally these can undergo malignant transformation to Wilms' tumor.
▶ Conditions associated with nephroblastomatosis include sporadic aniridia (which is rare but has the highest risk of Wilms' tumor), Beckwith-Wiedemann syndrome, hemihypertrophy, Drash syndrome (male pseudohermaphroditism/nephritis), and WAGR (Wilms', aniridia, genital anomalies and mental retardation).
▶ Nephrogenic rests are usually peripheral and triangular or pyramidal in contour. When they are round or large or have central necrosis, malignant transformation should be suspected. In the diffuse form, a hypo-enhancing rind is seen around the whole kidney. On ultrasound, nephrogenic rests are hypo- or isoechoic to cortex. CT and MR are much more sensitive for nephrogenic rests than is ultrasound. On CT, they enhance less than normal cortex, and on MR they appear homogeneous and iso- to hypointense on T1- and iso- to hypointense on T2-weighted images.

Next steps in management

Screening of patients with predisposing conditions consists of baseline CT or MR at 6 months of age and screening every 3 to 4 months thereafter with alternating ultrasound and MR exams until age 7 or 8 years.

Further reading

1. Lowe LH, Isuani BH, Heller RM, et al. Pediatric renal masses: Wilms tumor and beyond. Radiographics. 2000 Nov–Dec;20(6):1585–1603.
2. Smets AM, de Kraker J. Malignant tumours of the kidney: imaging strategy. Pediatr Radiol. 2010 Jun;40(6):1010–1018.

History

► 2-week-old boy with abnormal prenatal ultrasound.

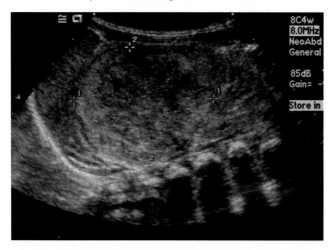

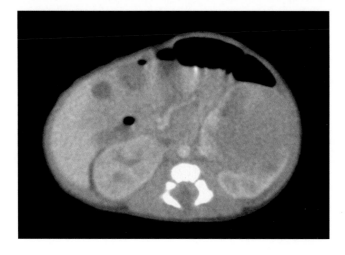

Case 56   Mesoblastic Nephroma

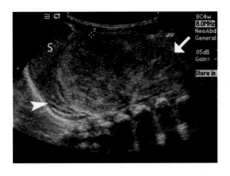
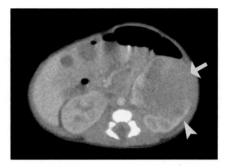

Findings

▶ Longitudinal ultrasound image (left) shows a mass (calipers) arising from the left kidney (arrow). Also noted are the normal adrenal gland (arrowhead) and spleen (S).

▶ Axial enhanced CT image (right) confirms the renal origin of the mass (arrow) with the claw sign (arrowhead).

Differential diagnosis

The most common renal tumor is Wilms' tumor, which has a very similar appearance, but Wilms' tumor is not a congenital tumor, so the most likely diagnosis is mesoblastic nephroma.

Teaching points

▶ Mesoblastic nephroma is a congenital renal tumor that is usually diagnosed by the age of 6 months. Most are incidental findings but patients may have hypertension or hypercalcemia.

▶ Histologically, there are two types: classic and cellular. The classic subtype occurs under the age of 3 months, has a benign course, and is predominantly solid on imaging without hemorrhage or necrosis. The cellular subtype occurs in slightly older infants and is typically larger at diagnosis. Hemorrhage and necrosis are common in the cellular subtype and the biologic behavior is more aggressive.

▶ On imaging, the tumor generally appears circumscribed, solid, and homogeneous and typically involves the renal sinus. Cystic areas of necrosis or old hemorrhage may also be noted. There are no imaging features that distinguish mesoblastic nephroma from Wilms' tumor, but the age of the patient is very suggestive.

▶ Recurrence and metastatic disease are rare, but patients with the cellular subtype should be followed for 1 year after resection.

Next steps in management

Nephrectomy is the treatment of choice. Wide margins are necessary as the tumor is histologically infiltrative.

Further reading

1. Lowe LH, Isuani BH, Heller RM, et al. Pediatric renal masses: Wilms tumor and beyond. Radiographics. 2000 Nov–Dec; 20(6):1585–1603.
2. Ahmed HU, Arya M, Levitt G, et al. Part I: Primary malignant non-Wilms' renal tumours in children. Lancet Oncol. 2007 Aug;8(8):730–737.

History

► 2-year-old boy with palpable left abdominal mass.

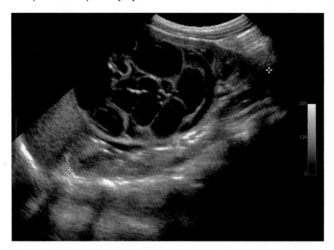

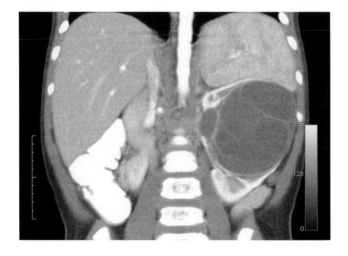

Case 57 Cystic Nephroma

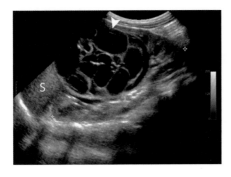 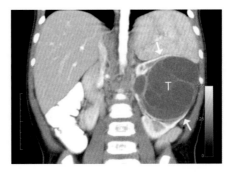

Findings

▶ Longitudinal ultrasound image (left) reveals a cystic mass (arrowhead) arising from the left kidney (calipers). (S = spleen)

▶ CT coronal reconstruction (right) shows the mass (T) is cystic with enhancement of only the walls and septa. The renal claw sign is noted (arrows).

Differential diagnosis

By far the most common renal tumor is Wilms' tumor, which may be cystic, but the differential for cystic renal masses includes multicystic dysplastic kidney (MCDK) and renal lymphoma, which may appear cystic on ultrasound. The finding of renal parenchyma around the mass excludes MCDK except the rare segmental type. Involvement of the kidney with lymphoma is usually a late finding when the diagnosis of lymphoma is well established.

Teaching points

▶ Multilocular cystic renal tumor represents two radiologically indistinguishable but histologically distinct tumors.
   ▪ Cystic nephroma—benign tumor with mature cells in the septa
   ▪ Cystic partially differentiated nephroblastoma (CPDN)—has blastemal cells in the septa and is part of the spectrum of nephroblastoma (Wilms' tumor)

▶ A small number of patients present with hematuria due to prolapse of the tumor into the renal collecting system.

▶ There is a bimodal age distribution—young boys and adult women.

▶ Cystic nephroma and CPDN are composed of cysts with septations of varying thickness with no round solid components. Only the walls and the septations enhance. The tumors may be seen filling the renal collecting system, a suggestive but uncommon finding.

▶ Metastatic disease has not been reported.

Next steps in management

Cystic nephroma and CPDN are not distinguishable preoperatively. Both are treated with complete resection. CPDN carries a risk of recurrence and these patients should be followed with imaging.

Further reading

1. Lowe LH, Isuani BH, Heller RM, et al. Pediatric renal masses: Wilms tumor and beyond. Radiographics. 2000 Nov–Dec; 20(6):1585–1603.
2. Silver IM, Boag AH, Soboleski DA. Best cases from the AFIP: Multilocular cystic renal tumor: cystic nephroma. Radiographics. 2008 Jul–Aug;28(4):1221–1226.

History

▶ 6-month-old with protuberant abdomen.

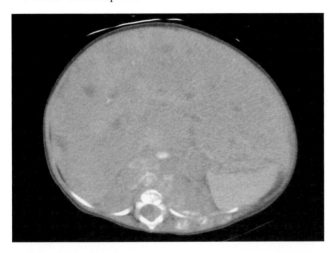

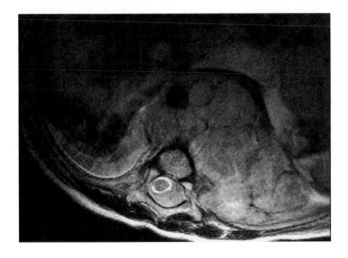

Case 58 Adrenal Neuroblastoma with Liver Metastases

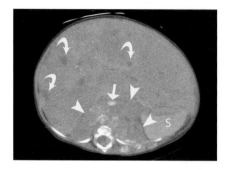 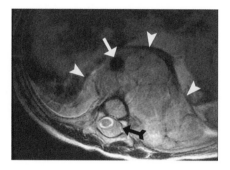

Findings

▶ Axial CT image (left) and axial T2-weighted MR images show partially calcified, T2-hyperintense mass (arrowheads) medial to the spleen (S), extending across midline behind the aorta (arrow). CT shows hypoattenuating liver nodules (curved arrows) and MR shows mass in the spinal canal (tailed arrow) deviating the spinal cord to the right.

Differential diagnosis

Adrenal tumors may originate in the cortex or the medulla. Medullary tumors include neuroblastoma and pheochromocytoma. Cortical tumors include adenomas and carcinomas. In the neonate, the main differential diagnostic consideration is adrenal hemorrhage. Because of the excellent prognosis for infants under age 1 year with neuroblastoma, close follow-up with ultrasound is safe. Hematomas will get smaller, while neuroblastoma will enlarge.

Teaching points

▶ Neuroblastoma is a tumor originating from neural crest tissue in the adrenal medulla and the sympathetic chain and the second most common abdominal malignancy. Other sites include the thorax, neck, and pelvis.
▶ Neuroblastoma and related tumors demonstrate a spectrum of differentiation. Least differentiated and most malignant is neuroblastoma. The median age at diagnosis is 22 months, although the tumor can be congenital. Ganglioneuroblastomas are less aggressive tumors in older children. Ganglioneuromas are benign and occur in adolescents and adults. Neuroblastomas demonstrate widely varied biologic activity. They may widely metastasize or they may spontaneously differentiate into benign tumors.
▶ Neuroblastomas in neonates tend to be predominantly cystic, while they are solid in older children.
▶ Spread is to adjacent lymph nodes, liver, and bones.
▶ Stage 4S disease is a special category that occurs in an infant under 1 year of age with a unilateral primary tumor and spread limited to liver, skin, and bone marrow. Though the disease may be extensive, the long-term prognosis is excellent.

Next steps in management

Diagnosis is made by demonstrating elevated urinary catecholamines and with tissue biopsy.

Further reading
1. Lonergan GJ, Schwab CM, Suarez ES, Carlson CL. Neuroblastoma, ganglioneuroblastoma, and ganglioneuroma: radiologic-pathologic correlation. Radiographics. 2002 Jul–Aug;22(4):911–934.
2. McHugh K. Renal and adrenal tumours in children. Cancer Imaging. 2007 Mar 5;7:41–51.

History

▶ 1-day-old with birth asphyxia.

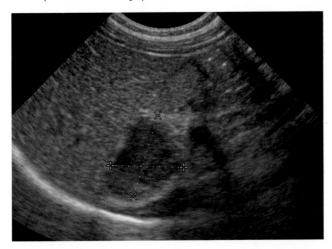

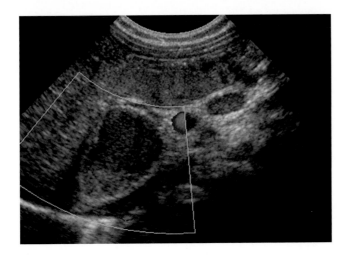

Case 59 Adrenal Hemorrhage

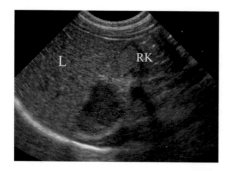 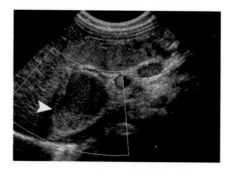

Findings

▶ Longitudinal ultrasound image (left) shows a triangular, hypoechoic mass in the right renal fossa (calipers). (L = liver, RK = right kidney)

▶ Color Doppler image (right) shows no flow in the mass and the appearance of a fluid level or hematocrit (arrowhead).

Differential diagnosis

Neonatal hypoechoic renal mass may also represent a cystic congenital neuroblastoma. There is no specific radiographic appearance for adrenal hemorrhage. Both conditions may be diagnosed prenatally and may be bilateral. The diagnosis of adrenal hemorrhage is suggested by a history of perinatal stress. The additional finding of ipsilateral renal vein thrombosis supports adrenal hemorrhage. The finding of Doppler flow within the lesion or liver metastases indicates neuroblastoma.

Teaching points

▶ Macrosomic infants or infants with maternal diabetes are at risk. Most hemorrhages occur on the right side.

▶ Very large hemorrhages are round and the normal adrenal gland is not identified. Smaller hemorrhages are triangular. Large hemorrhages may extend into the retroperitoneum and scrotum.

▶ The appearance on ultrasound depends on the timing of the exam. Initially, the hemorrhage is usually of mixed echogenicity, evolving to a hypo- or anechoic appearance of old blood products. This change occurs in a week or so. During this time, the hematoma becomes smaller and begins to calcify.

▶ Adrenal calcifications due to prior hemorrhage may be found on radiographs in an older child. If there is a history of perinatal stress and the calcification conforms to a normal adrenal shape, no further imaging is necessary. Otherwise, ultrasound is indicated to exclude a mass.

Next steps in management

There are no specific findings for adrenal hemorrhage, but the hemorrhage will evolve within a week or two, and the diagnosis is confirmed on close interval follow-up.

Further reading

1. Bergami G, Malena S, Demario M, Fariello G. Sonographic follow-up of neonatal adrenal hemorrhage: fourteen case reports. Radiol Med. 1990;79:474–478.
2. Eo H, Kim JH, Jang KM, et al. Comparison of clinic-radiologic features between congenital cystic neuroblastoma and neonatal adrenal hemorrhagic pseudocyst. Korean J Radiol. 2011 Jan;12(1):52–58.

History

▶ Newborn boy with abnormal prenatal ultrasound.

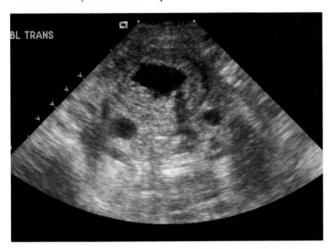

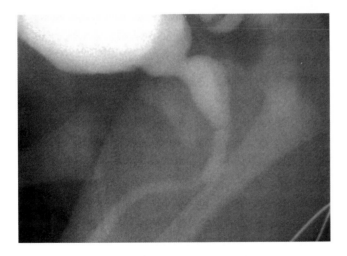

Case 60 Posterior Urethral Valves (PUV)

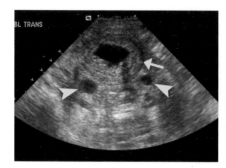 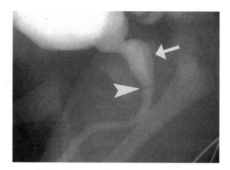

Findings

▸ Transverse ultrasound image (left) shows a markedly thickened and irregular bladder wall (arrow) and dilated distal ureters (arrowheads).

▸ Lateral voiding image from a voiding cystourethrogram (VCUG) demonstrates dilation of the posterior urethra (arrow) and an obstructing membrane (arrowhead).

Differential diagnosis

Hydronephrosis could also be related to prune belly or Eagle-Barrett syndrome. In most cases of prune belly, the bladder is large and floppy, but in the severe form, there is an anatomic obstruction and a trabeculated bladder as seen in PUV. Also, the posterior urethra may be dilated in Eagle-Barrett syndrome, but there is no valve.

Teaching points

▸ PUV represent remnants of the mesonephric ducts that form an obstruction to urine flow. Autopsy studies have shown that the obstruction is an oblique membrane rather than valves, so an alternative term, congenital obstructive posterior membrane (COPUM), has been proposed.

▸ Most present early in infancy with UTI due to stasis or poor urinary stream or are prenatally diagnosed.

▸ The finding of secondary signs of obstruction, including the thick-walled, trabeculated bladder, and the dilated posterior urethra above the membrane, are helpful in distinguishing the valves from the normal plicae collicularis.

▸ Bilateral hydronephrosis in a newborn boy is considered due to PUV until proved otherwise, but only 50% of patients with PUV have bilateral hydronephrosis. The rest have unilateral or no hydronephrosis.

▸ In utero obstruction causes renal dysplasia and the overall prognosis depends on the degree of dysplasia. Factors that protect one or both kidneys reduce the pressure transmitted from the bladder to the kidney(s) and include a large bladder, a large bladder or calyceal diverticulum, absence of vesicoureteral reflux (hydronephrosis), and forniceal rupture leading to urinary ascites.

Next steps in management

The VCUG is diagnostic and the treatment is surgical.

Further Reading

1. Levin TL, Han B, Little BP. Congenital anomalies of the male urethra.Pediatr Radiol. 2007 Sep;37(9):851–862.
2. Mercado-Deane MG, Beeson JE, John SD. US of renal insufficiency in neonates. Radiographics. 2002 Nov–Dec;22(6): 1429–1438.

History

▶ 4-year-old boy with left flank pain.

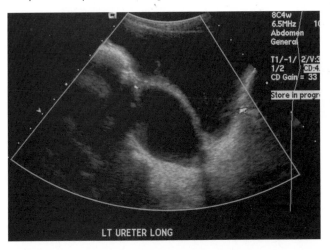

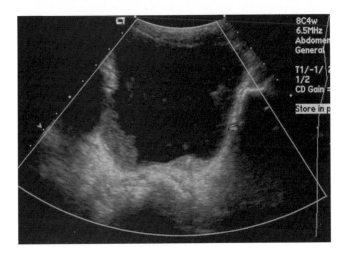

Case 61   Primary Megaureter with Stone

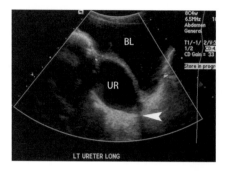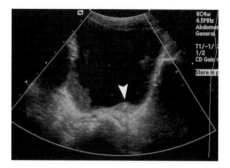

Findings

▶ Longitudinal ultrasound image (left) reveals a markedly dilated ureter (UR) behind the bladder (BL) with a small focus of acoustic shadowing (arrowhead).

▶ Transverse image of the bladder (right) shows a tiny echogenic focus with posterior shadowing representing a stone (arrowhead).

Differential diagnosis

Dilation of the ureter may be due to vesicoureteric reflux, obstruction, or primary megaureter. In young children, the most common cause is reflux, but in this case a stone is visualized. The degree of dilation of the ureter is too great to be explained by obstruction due to ureterolith alone. Rather than the cause of dilation, the stone is the result of primary megaureter with stasis leading to stone formation.

Teaching points

▶ The term "primary megaureter" describes ureteral dilation due to an idiopathic congenital abnormality of the ureterovesical junction. These conditions may be further categorized as obstructed, refluxing, or nonrefluxing, nonobstructed primary megaureter.

▶ Obstructed primary megaureter is a functional obstruction with a short aperistaltic segment of distal ureter with a normal ureteral insertion analogous to Hirschsprung disease of the GI tract. As in Hirschsprung disease, it is the normal proximal ureter that becomes dilated due to the distal obstruction, while the aperistaltic segment maintains a normal caliber. Nonrefluxing, nonobstructed primary megaureter is idiopathic, but one theory is that it represents an ultra-short form of obstructed primary megaureter.

▶ Urine stasis predisposes to infection and stone formation. The stone lodges in the nondilated, aperistaltic segment.

Next steps in management

Asymptomatic patients are followed with ultrasound to ensure that the condition is not worsening. Most remain stable. Symptomatic patients or those with severe or worsening dilation are treated with surgery.

Further reading

1. Berrocal T, López-Pereira P, Arjonilla A, Gutiérrez J. Anomalies of the distal ureter, bladder, and urethra in children: embryologic, radiologic, and pathologic features. Radiographics. 2002 Sep–Oct;22(5):1139–1164.
2. Ebel KD. Uroradiology in the fetus and newborn: diagnosis and follow-up of congenital obstruction of the urinary tract. Pediatr Radiol. 1998 Aug;28(8):630–635.

History

▸ 1-week-old boy with UTI.

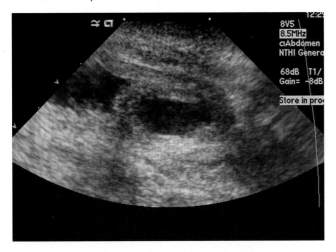

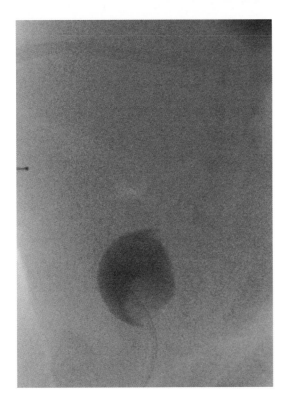

Case 62 Ureterocele

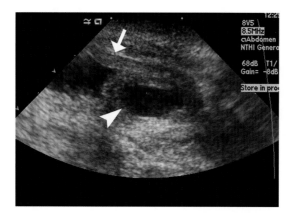 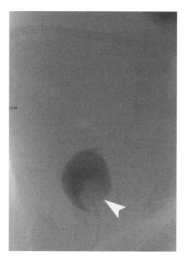

Findings

▸ Longitudinal ultrasound image (left) shows a cyst (arrowhead) in the bladder. Arrow indicates bladder wall.
▸ Early-filling view from a voiding cystourethrogram (VCUG) shows a smooth-walled filling defect (arrowhead).

Differential diagnosis

Foreign objects, such as Foley catheter balloons, may also cause bladder filling defects but are uncommon.

Teaching points

▸ A ureterocele is a dilation of the distal ureter, usually due to ureterovesical junction (UVJ) obstruction, which invaginates into the bladder.
▸ Ureteroceles may be ectopic (associated with an ectopic ureter) or simple. Ectopic ureteroceles are more common in girls with duplex kidneys. These are often large and may cause obstruction of the bladder outlet or the contralateral UVJ or they may herniate through the urethra and present as an interlabial mass.
▸ Ureteroceles in boys are often small and asymptomatic. These have the appearance of a cobra head or spring onion. When there is contrast in the distal ureter and the bladder, there is a lucent rim or halo around the ureterocele as it is lined by two layers of urothelium—that of the bladder and that of the ureter.
▸ Ureteroceles are dynamic in size and shape. With bladder filling, they become less apparent, in part due to obscuration by dense contrast, but also due to change in relative pressure in the bladder compared to the ureterocele. As the bladder fills, the pressure in the bladder exceeds that in the ureterocele and the ureterocele is compressed. With further filling, the ureterocele may even evert and mimic the appearance of a bladder diverticulum. For these reasons, ureteroceles are best visualized on early-filling views.

Next steps in management

Small, incidental ureteroceles are not treated. Large, symptomatic ureteroceles are treated with cystoscopic marsupialization.

Further reading

1. Berrocal T, López-Pereira P, Arjonilla A, Gutiérrez J. Anomalies of the distal ureter, bladder, and urethra in children: embryologic, radiologic and pathologic features. Radiographics. 2002 Sep–Oct;22(5):1139–1164.
2. Fernbach SK, Feinstein KA, Schmidt MB. Pediatric voiding cystourethrography: a pictoral guide. Radiographics. 2000 Jan–Feb;20(1):155–168.

History

▶ 8-day-old boy with persistently draining umbilicus.

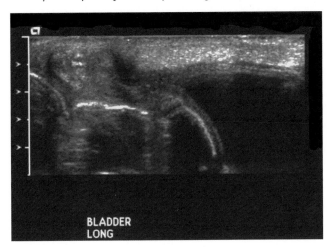

Case 63 Patent Urachus

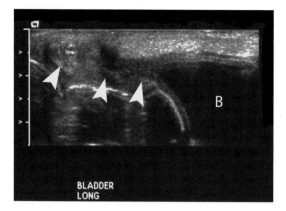

Findings

▶ Longitudinal ultrasound image of the anterior abdominal wall shows a tubular structure (arrowheads) connecting the anterior superior bladder (B) to the umbilicus.

Differential diagnosis

Drainage from the urachus may be due to urachal remnant, which connects to the bladder, or to a remnant of the omphalomesenteric or vitelline duct, which connects to the intestine.

Teaching points

▶ There are four types of urachal anomalies:
- Patent urachus—open at both ends
- Urachal sinus—closed on the bladder end
- Urachal diverticulum—closed at the umbilical end
- Urachal cyst—closed at both ends with fluid trapped between

▶ Patients with patent urachus are diagnosed in the neonatal period due to persistent leakage of urine from the urachus. The other anomalies are usually asymptomatic but may produce symptoms if they become infected.

▶ Patent urachus and urachal diverticulum are seen in patients with urethral obstruction such as those with posterior urethral valves, urethral atresia/stenosis, or Eagle-Barrett syndrome.

▶ Urachal anomalies are well evaluated with ultrasound, particularly in the sagittal plane. The urachal sinus appears as a tubular structure that connects only to the umbilicus. The urachal diverticulum appears as an outpouching of the anterior superior aspect of the bladder. The urachal cyst is a midline cyst between the bladder and umbilicus. These are commonly infected at the time of diagnosis. The diagnosis of patent urachus can be confirmed with cystography or fistulography.

▶ A late complication of urachal remnant is the development of adenocarcinoma of the urachus. Like other adenocarcinomas, urachal carcinoma may produce psammomatous calcifications that are visible on CT.

Next steps in management

Small urachal anomalies found in the perinatal period may resolve on follow-up by age 6 months. Otherwise treatment is minimally invasive surgery.

Further reading

1. Yu JS, Kim KW, Lee HJ, et al. Urachal remnant diseases: spectrum of CT and US findings. Radiographics. 2001;21(2): 451–461.
2. Galati V, Donovan B, Ramji F, et al. Management of urachal remnants in early childhood. J Urol. 2008;180(4 Suppl): 1824–1826.

History

▶ 5-year-old with hematuria.

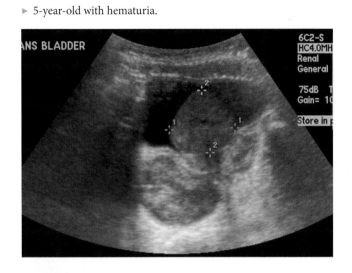

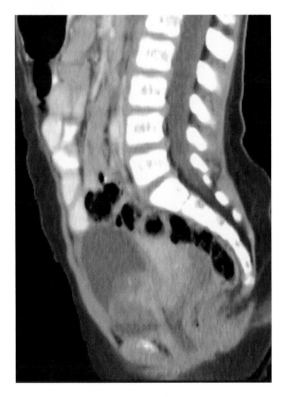

Case 64   Vaginal Rhabdomyosarcoma with Bladder Invasion

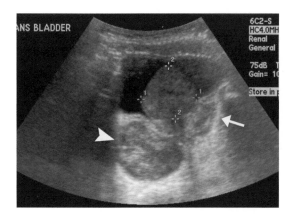
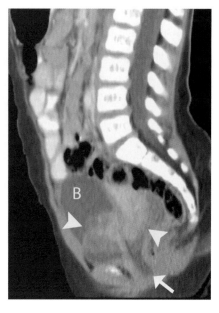

Findings

▶ Transverse ultrasound image of the bladder shows a polypoid posterior bladder mass (calipers) and a mass posterior to the bladder (arrowhead). The arrow indicates the uterus.

▶ Sagittal CT reformat shows the mass (arrowheads) in the vagina (arrow) and bladder (B).

Differential diagnosis

If the mass were in only the bladder or the vagina and did not enhance it could represent a hematoma. The mass may have originated from the bladder or the vagina. In either case, the most likely diagnosis is rhabdomyosarcoma. If the mass appeared to arise from the presacral space, neuroblastoma and teratoma should be considered.

Teaching points

▶ Rhabdomyosarcoma is the most common tumor arising in the pelvis. In girls it generally arises from the vagina, cervix, uterus, or the trigone of the bladder. In boys, rhabdomyosarcoma typically arises from the prostate or scrotum.

▶ Pelvic rhabdomyosarcoma is usually of the botryoid or embryonal type.

▶ On imaging studies the tumor appears as a somewhat heterogeneous soft tissue mass, frequently with lobulated margins. In the bladder the mass may appear polypoid.

▶ Spread of disease is to pelvic lymph nodes, liver, lung, and bone.

Next steps in management

Imaging of the chest, abdomen, and pelvis with CT or MR is indicated for staging. Pelvic MR is superior to CT in the evaluation for local spread. Bone scintigraphy is indicated to evaluate for bony metastases.

Further reading

1. Argons GA, Wagner BJ, Lonergan GJ, Dickey GE, Kaufman MS. Genitourinary rhabdomyosarcoma in children: radiologic-pathologic correlation. Radiographics. 1997;17:919–937.
2. Fletcher BD, Kaste SC. Magnetic resonance imaging for diagnosis and follow-up of genitourinary, pelvic, and perineal rhabdomyosarcoma. Urol Radiol. 1992;14:262–272.

History

▶ 7-month-old with UTI.

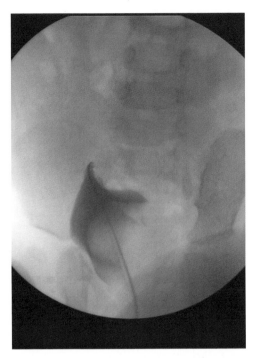

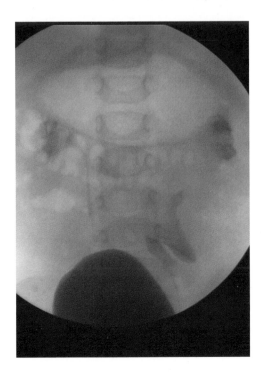

Case 65   Vesicureteral Reflux into Lower Pole of Duplex Kidneys with Left Upper Pole Ureterocele

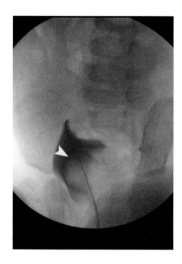 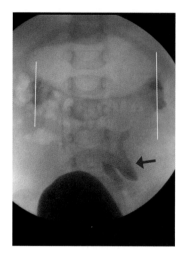

Findings

▸ Oblique early-filling view from a voiding cystourethrogram (VCUG) shows a round, leftward filling defect in the bladder (arrowhead), representing a ureterocele.

▸ AP image shows bilateral grade II vesicoureteral reflux (VUR) and abnormal, vertical axis of the intrarenal collecting systems (white lines), indicating duplex kidneys. Arrow indicates left ureter.

Teaching points

▸ VUR is usually a primary abnormality of the ureterovesical junction (UVJ), which is familial and usually resolves with advancing age, so that it is much less common after the age of 6 years. On oblique images from a VCUG, the UVJ appears normal. VUR may also be secondary to bladder outlet obstruction or abnormal ureteral insertion.

▸ Current indications for VCUG or ultrasound with intravesical contrast (urosonography) include febrile UTI, first UTI in a boy or recurrent UTI in a girl under the age of 6 years, solitary functioning kidney, abnormal ultrasound, neurogenic bladder, and following ureteral reimplantation.

▸ Renal ultrasound is normal in 75% of patients with VUR. If abnormal, the ultrasound will show hydronephrosis. In young children, the most common cause of hydronephrosis is VUR. The purpose of the US is to evaluate for renal scarring.

▸ Evaluation of pediatric UTI is evolving. Ongoing research studies are focusing on changing the emphasis to primarily evaluating for renal scarring with renal cortical scintigraphy rather than starting with cystourethrography to evaluate for reflux.

Next steps in management

Primary VUR is treated with antibiotic prophylaxis. Follow-up radionuclide cystography is performed annually. If the condition worsens or fails to resolve or if renal scarring is found, then surgical options are ureteral reimplantation or cystoscopic subureteric injection of Deflux.

Further reading

1. American Academy of Pediatrics Committee on Quality Improvement Subcommittee on Urinary Tract Infection. Practice parameter: the diagnosis, treatment and evaluation of the initial urinary tract infection in febrile infants and young children. Pediatrics 1999;103:842–852.
2. Lim R. Vesicoureteral reflux and urinary tract infection: evolving practices and current controversies in pediatric imaging. AJR Am J Roentgenol. 2009 May;192(5):1197–1208.

History

▶ 1-year-old with UTI.

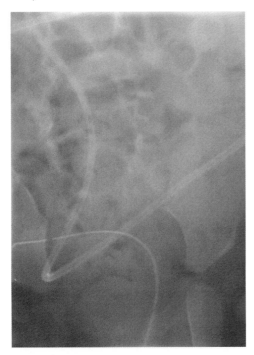

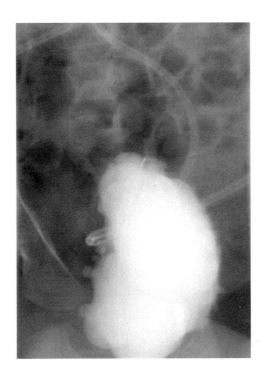

Case 66 Neurogenic Bladder/Spinal Dysraphism

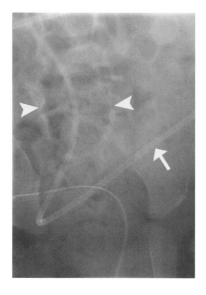 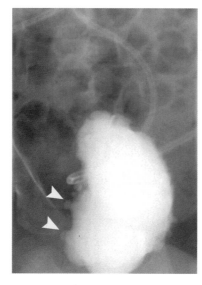

Findings

▶ AP scout image from a voiding cystourethrogram (VCUG) shows spinal dysraphism with splaying of the pedicles of the sacral spine (arrowheads) and a ventriculoperitoneal (VP) shunt (arrow).

▶ Oblique image from VCUG shows that the bladder configuration is taller than wide and the wall is irregular with multiple diverticula (arrowheads).

Differential diagnosis

This patient with a VP shunt has a known diagnosis of myelomeningocele (open dysraphism), but some patients with spinal dysraphism have a skin-covered defect (closed dysraphism), usually do not have significant hydrocephalus, and often can walk. All patients with dysraphism have neurogenic bladder. Patients with sacral agenesis can also have neurogenic bladder. In these cases, examination of the scout radiograph for lumbosacral anomalies may be the first indication of the diagnosis of an underlying neurologic cause for UTI. Additionally, these patients have constipation. A neurologic cause should be suspected in patients with recurrent UTI and constipation.

Teaching points

▶ On VCUG, the bladder appears as in this case. Also, the bladder neck will be inappropriately funnel-shaped when the bladder is filling. Usually these patients cannot void. The contrast is drained via the catheter. They also usually cannot feel that the bladder is full, so the end point of the exam is overflow incontinence.

▶ These patients are at lifelong risk of developing vesicoureteral reflux (VUR) and are screened with VCUG biennially. If left untreated, the VUR could lead to renal insufficiency.

Next steps in management

If the diagnosis was previously unknown, spinal MRI is indicated. If the bladder becomes small and non-compliant due to stasis and recurrent infections, an orthotopic neobladder may be created with small bowel or autologous bladder cells.

Further reading

1. Fotter R. Neurogenic bladder in infants and children—a new challenge for the radiologist. Abdom Imaging. 1996 Nov–Dec; 21(6):534–540.
2. Blane CE, Zerin JM, Bloom DA. Bladder diverticula in children. Radiology. 1994 Mar;190(3):695–697.

History

▶ Newborn boy with no palpable left testis in the scrotum.

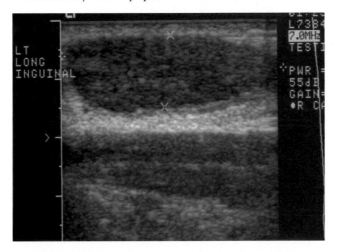

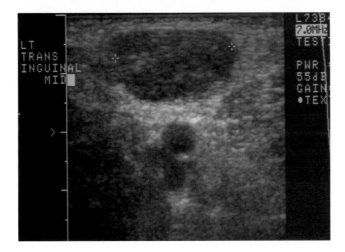

Case 67   Undescended Testis

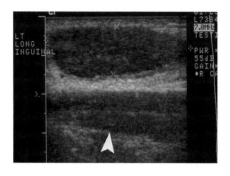 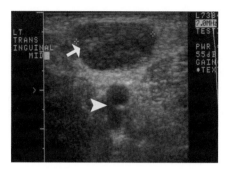

Findings

▶ Longitudinal (left) and transverse (right) ultrasound image of the left inguinal region shows an ovoid hypoechoic mass (calipers) with a echogenic fan-like mediastinum testis (arrow). This testis is superficial to the femoral vessels (arrowhead).

Differential diagnosis

Inguinal mass could also represent inguinal hernia, which may coexist with cryptorchidism. Bilateral cryptorchidism could be a manifestation of an intersex state.

Teaching points

▶ Normally the testes descend into the scrotum by the third trimester, but 4% of newborn boys have one or more undescended testes. Most will descend into the scrotum by age 1 year. Approximately a third of cases are bilateral.

▶ Most undescended testes are located in the inguinal canal, and are frequently palpable in the inguinal canal. The inguinal regions are well evaluated with ultrasound. The testis may be distinguished by its homogeneous appearance, ovoid shape, and its linear, echogenic mediastinum testis.

▶ If the testis is nonpalpable and not found in the inguinal canal, it may be undescended or ectopic in the abdomen or pelvis. MRI may be useful to localize abdominal or pelvic testes.

▶ Complications include infertility and malignant transformation to seminoma or other germ cell tumor in adulthood.

Next steps in management

Treatment is orchiopexy at age 1 year.

Further reading

1. Christensen JD, Dogra VS. The undescended testis. Semin Ultrasound CT MR. 2007 Aug;28:307–316.
2. Frush DP, Sheldon CA. Diagnostic imaging for pediatric scrotal disorders. Radiographics. 1998 Jul–Aug;18:969–985.

History

▶ Newborn boy with enlarged, discolored left testicle.

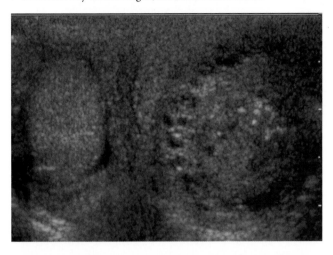

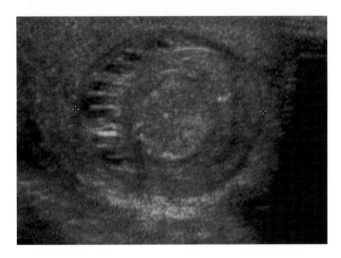

Case 68   In Utero Testicular Torsion

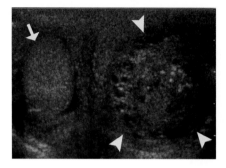 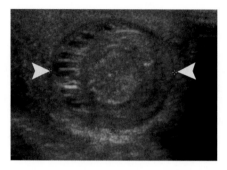

Findings

▶ Transverse ultrasound image of both testes (left) and of left testis (right) show a normal right testis (arrow) and an enlarged heterogeneous left testicle (arrowheads) with small hyperechoic foci.

Differential diagnosis

The differential diagnosis of acute scrotum in a boy includes torsion of the appendix testis or appendix epididymis, epididymo-orchitis, and incarcerated inguinal hernia. In a neonate, the differential of an enlarged testis includes inguinal hernia, hydrocele, hematocele, and meconium periorchitis.

Teaching points

▶ Testicular torsion most commonly occurs in the peripubertal and perinatal periods.
▶ In peripubertal boys, as in young adults, the torsion is intravaginal. The tunica vaginalis covers the testis and most of the epididymis. When the tunica extends over the spermatic cord, these structures are allowed to freely twist within the tunica. This is the "bell clapper" deformity.
▶ On ultrasound, the torsed testicle may be slightly hypoechoic and enlarged. There is decreased color-flow compared to the opposite testicle. Pulse-wave Doppler evaluation shows decreased diastolic flow. Torsion can be intermittent, so the finding of flow to the testis does not exclude torsion, and the spermatic cord should be evaluated for torsion.
▶ In perinatal cases, the torsion is extravaginal and results from deficient attachment of the tunica vaginalis to the scrotal wall, allowing the testicle, epididymis, and the tunica itself to twist. This may occur antenatally.
▶ On ultrasound, the sequela of in utero torsion is a small, heterogeneously hypoechoic testis that may have a calcified rim.

Next steps in management

Surgical detorsion of the testis within 6 hours is associated with a high likelihood of salvageability. In the case of in utero torsion, the involved testis is not likely to be salvageable, but orchiopexy of the other testis prevents the risk of anorchia.

Further reading

1. Traubici J, Daneman A, Navarro O, et al. Testicular torsion in neonates and infants: sonographic features in 30 patients. AJR Am J Roentgenol. 2003;180:1143–1144.
2. Frush DP, Sheldon CA. Diagnostic imaging for pediatric scrotal disorders. Radiographics. 1998 Jul–Aug;18:969–985.

History

▶ 17-year-old with testicular mass.

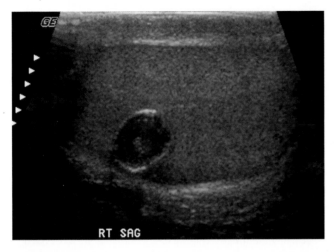

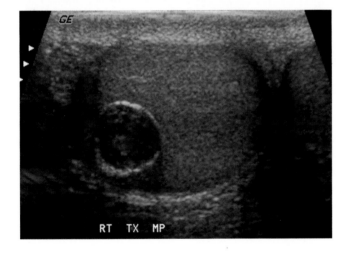

Case 69   Epidermoid Cyst

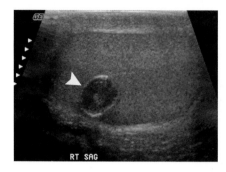 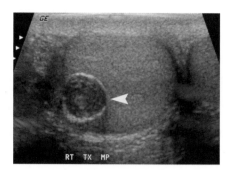

Findings

▶ Longitudinal (left) and transverse (right) ultrasound images reveal a well-circumscribed hypoechoic lesion in the right testicle with echogenic margin and internal echoes in a whorled pattern (arrowhead).

Differential diagnosis

Intratesticular lesions are more likely to be malignant than extratesticular lesions, but are more likely benign in a child than in an adult. Scrotal rhabdomyosarcoma may occur in children. The differential diagnosis for intratesticular tumors in young children is different than in adults. In adults and adolescents, the most common malignancies are seminomas, which are rare prior to puberty. In boys, the most common germ cell tumor is the yolk sac tumor. Benign lesions include mature teratoma and epidermoid. Mature teratoma contains fat and calcifications. Epidermoid cyst is distinguished by the whorled or lamellated appearance of the layers of keratin.

Teaching points

▶ Most intratesticular neoplasms in children are germ cell tumors. Yolk sac tumor (endodermal sinus tumor) peaks at 2 years of age and causes elevation of the serum alpha-fetoprotein (AFP) level. Elevated serum hCG levels occur in embryonal cell carcinoma and teratocarcinoma, which rarely occur prior to puberty. The ultrasound appearance is generally nonspecific.

▶ Mature teratoma is the most common benign testicular tumor of young children.

▶ Less common intratesticular tumors are stromal tumors—Leydig and Sertoli cell tumors, which may present with hormonal syndromes.
  ▪ Leydig cell tumor—testosterone—precocious puberty
  ▪ Sertoli cell tumor—estrogens—gynecomastia

▶ Because of the blood–gonad barrier, the testes may act as a sanctuary for leukemic cells. Leukemic testicular infiltrates are typically bilateral.

▶ Spread of malignant tumors is to retroperitoneal and regional lymph nodes, lung, and brain.

Next steps in management

Imaging with CT or MR for abdominopelvic spread and lung metastases is indicated. If the tumor appears typical of teratoma or epidermoid and tumor markers are negative, then testicle-sparing surgery is possible.

Further reading

1. Frush DP, Sheldon CA. Diagnostic imaging for pediatric scrotal disorders. Radiographics. 1998 Jul–Aug;18:969–985.
2. Carkaci S, Ozkan E, Lane D, Yang WT. Scrotal sonography revisted. J Clin Ultrasound. 2010 Jan;38(1):21–37.

History

▶ 11-year-old with pelvic pain.

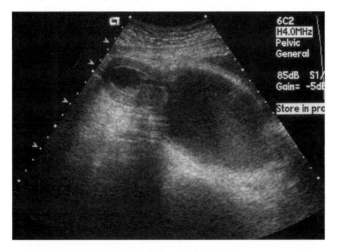

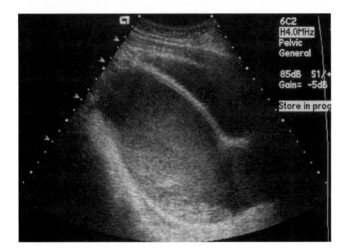

Case 70 Hematometrocolpos due to Imperforate Hymen

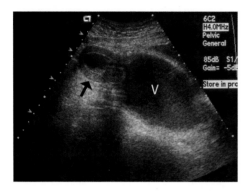 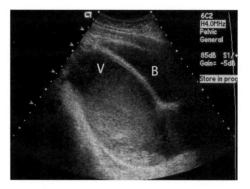

Findings

▶ Longitudinal ultrasound images (right caudal to left) show a markedly dilated vagina (V) behind the bladder (B) filled with echogenic debris. The endometrial cavity of the uterus (arrow) is also dilated.

Differential diagnosis

Demonstration of the relationship of the dilated tubular structure to the uterus confirms the diagnosis of hydro- or hematocolpos.

Teaching points

▶ Hydrocolpos is dilation of the vagina with simple fluid and hematocolpos is dilation with echogenic blood. If the endometrial canal is also dilated, then the condition is called hematometrocolpos.

▶ Patients may present with cyclical pelvic pain and/or delayed menarche. The condition may occur in neonates due to stimulation of secretions by maternal hormones.

▶ Underlying causes include the following:
  ▪ Imperforate hymen—treated with an outpatient procedure
  ▪ Vaginal atresia or stenosis
    ◆ Associated with other GU and GI anomalies
    ◆ Requires more extensive surgery
  ▪ Imperforate vagina—fistula to urethra seen on voiding cystourethrogram

Next steps in management

Physical exam may differentiate underlying causes. In vaginal atresia, a search for other anomalies with ultrasound is warranted.

Further reading

1. López C, Balogun M, Ganesan R, Olliff JF. MRI of vaginal conditions. Clin Radiol. 2005 Jun;60(6):648–662.
2. Teele RL, Share JC. Ultrasonography of the female pelvis in childhood and adolescence. Radiol Clin North Am. 1992 Jul;30(4):743–758.

History

▶ 16-year-old with primary amenorrhea.

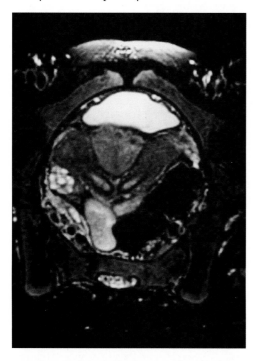

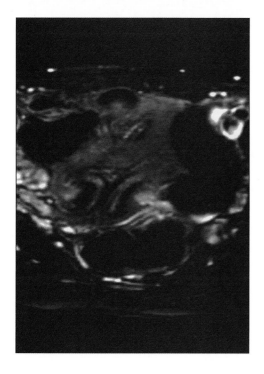

Case 71 Uterine Didelphys

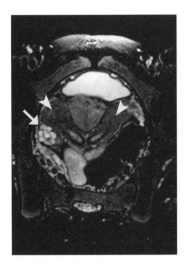 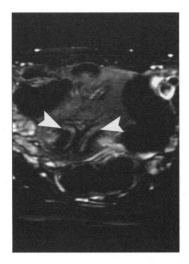

Findings

▸ Axial T2-weighted MR image (left) shows two separated uterine horns (arrowheads) with central cervices. The right ovary is seen (arrow).

▸ Coronal T2-weighted image (right) shows two parallel uterine cervices (arrowheads).

Differential diagnosis

Bicornuate bicollis uterus has similar features but wide separation of the uterine horns, and duplication of the upper vagina distinguishes uterine didelphys.

Teaching points

▸ Embryologically the uterus and upper third of the vagina develop from two paramesonephric or müllerian ducts. Normally, the caudal portions of the müllerian ducts fuse and the midline septum is resorbed. Complete failure of fusion results in uterine didelphys, in which there are two widely separated uterine horns, two cervices, and a vertical septum in the upper third of the vagina.

▸ The spectrum of fusion anomalies also includes bicornuate bicollis, in which there are two uterine horns and a septum extending through the cervix; bicornuate unicollis; and septate uterus, in which complete fusion occurs but there is failure of resorption of the midline septum. In the last, the upper fundal contour is convex.

▸ Failure of complete development of one müllerian duct results in a unicornuate uterus. If there is partial development, a rudimentary horn may be found.

▸ Uterine didelphys is asymptomatic unless one side is obstructed. This results in hematometrocolpos at menarche, which may obstruct the other side.

▸ Uterine fusion anomalies are associated with renal anomalies, including agenesis, ectopia, and dysgenesis. In unicornuate uterus with renal agenesis, the absent or rudimentary horn is ipsilateral to the renal agenesis. In uterine didelphys, one hemivagina may be obstructed. If there is coexisting renal agenesis, it is ipsilateral to the obstruction.

▸ Uterine anomalies are associated with early pregnancy losses and premature deliveries.

Next steps in management

If renal agenesis is discovered on imaging, uterine fusion anomaly should be sought and vice versa.

Further reading

1. Saleem SN. MR diagnosis of uterovaginal anomalies: current state of the art. Radiographics. 2003 Sep–Oct;23(5):e13.
2. Troiano RN, McCarthy SM. Mullerian duct anomalies: imaging and clinical issues. Radiology. 2004;233:19–34.

History

▶ 10-year-old boy with precocious puberty. First image is the right testis and second is the left.

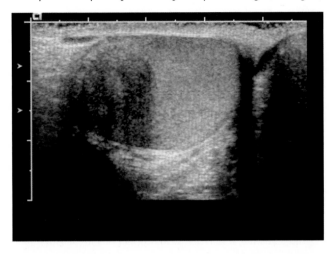

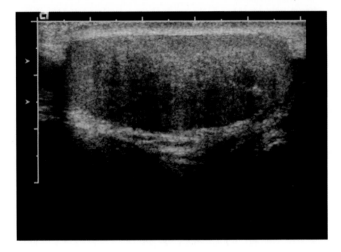

Case 72 Testicular Adrenal Rests/Congenital Adrenal Hyperplasia

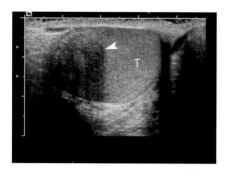 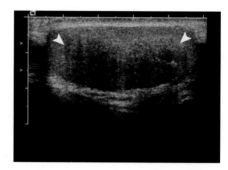

Findings

▶ Transverse ultrasound image (left) of the right testis (T) and longitudinal image of the left testis (right) show bilateral hypoechoic, shadowing foci in the region of the mediastinum testis (arrowheads).

Differential diagnosis

The fact that the condition is bilateral narrows the differential to testicular tumor of adrenogenital syndrome (adrenal rests), leukemia/lymphoma, or metastatic disease.

Teaching points

▶ Congenital adrenal hyperplasia (CAH) is an autosomal recessive deficiency of an adrenocortical enzyme, usually 21-hydroxylase, leading to underproduction of cortisol and aldosterone. Cortisol deficiency causes overproduction of adrenocorticotropic hormone (ACTH), which in turn causes hyperplasia of the adrenal glands and adrenal rest tissue in the testes.

▶ Testicular masses are seen in patients with inadequate glucocorticoid replacement therapy, leading to oversecretion of ACTH. Consequent overproduction of androgen precursors may lead to precocious puberty in boys.

▶ Ultrasound reveals bilateral hypoechoic testicular masses. These masses do not distort the outer contour of the testis, but the volume of the testes is frequently mildly increased. The masses frequently surround the echogenic mediastinum testis or occur laterally in the region of the mediastinum testis without a visible echogenic stripe in the center. Posterior acoustic shadowing may be noted, particularly with large masses.

▶ MR also shows bilateral peripheral masses that are iso- to slightly hyperintense to adjacent testicular parenchyma on T1-weighted images and hypointense on T2-weighted images. Most enhance with gadolinium.

▶ Ultrasound and MR are equally sensitive.

Next steps in management

Testicular tumors in CAH are treated with more aggressive hormonal therapy, and follow-up ultrasound is used to confirm regression of the masses.

Further reading

1. Avila NA, Premkumar A, Shawker TH, et al. Testicular adrenal rest tissue in congenital adrenal hyperplasia: findings at gray-scale and color Doppler US. Radiology. 1996 Jan;198(1):99–104.
2. Avila NA, Premkumar A, Merke DP. Testicular adrenal rest tissue in congenital adrenal hyperplasia: comparison of MR imaging and sonographic findings. AJR Am J Roentgenol. 1999 Apr;172(4):1003–1006.

History

▶ 4-year-old girl with right lower quadrant pain. First image is midline and second is on the left.

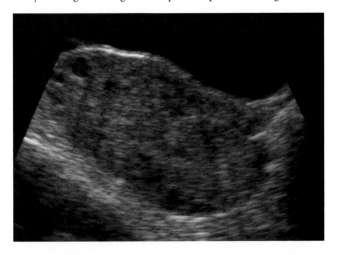

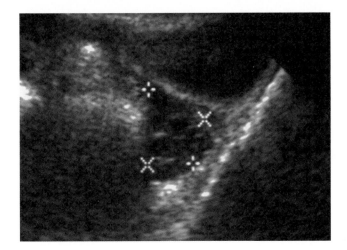

Case 73 Early Right Ovarian Torsion

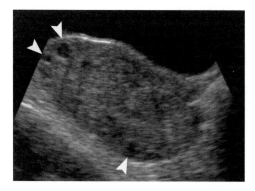 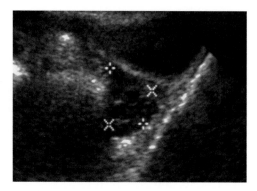

Findings

► Longitudinal transvesical ultrasound image of the right ovary (left) demonstrates that the ovary is enlarged and the follicles are distributed at the periphery (arrowheads).

► Comparison transverse image of the left ovary (right) shows normal size and diffuse distribution of the small follicles.

Differential diagnosis

The differential of right lower quadrant pain in a child includes appendicitis, epiploic appendagitis, and pyelonephritis.

Teaching points

► Torsion of the ovary is usually due to the presence of a large cyst or mass within the ovary. Torsion of a normal ovary may occur in young girls (4–6 years of age).

► As with testicular torsion, prior history of similar painful episodes is frequently elicited.

► The demonstration of Doppler flow to the gonad is much less meaningful in girls than in boys and in women, because of the increased distance between the transducer and the ovary. In virginal girls, endovaginal ultrasound is not performed.

► Much more helpful in the evaluation of suspected ovarian torsion is the appearance of the ovary. The torsed ovary is enlarged compared to its mate, and tends to be located in the midline posterior to the uterus.

► In early torsion, the venous and lymphatic drainage is occluded while the arterial flow is initially maintained. This causes the enlargement as edematous fluid accumulates in the center of the ovary, pushing the follicles to the periphery. The edema increases the resistance to arterial inflow, so the spectral waveform changes from low resistance to higher resistance.

► If the torsion persists, arterial inflow will be compromised and no flow is detected. The ovary becomes hemorrhagic and infarcted and appears heterogeneously hypoechoic.

Next steps in management

In early torsion, urgent surgery is required.

Further reading

1. Ratani RS, Cohen HL, Fiore E. Pediatric gynecologic ultrasound. Ultrasound Q. 2004 Sep;20(3):127–139.
2. Garel L, Dubois J, Grignon A, et al. US of the pediatric female pelvis: a clinical perspective. Radiographics. 2001 Nov–Dec;21(6):1393–1407.

History

▶ Prenatal ultrasound of female fetus at 35 weeks gestation.

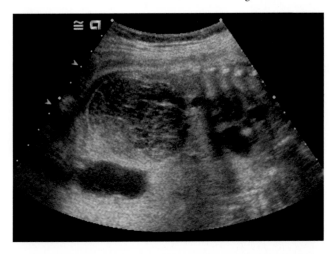

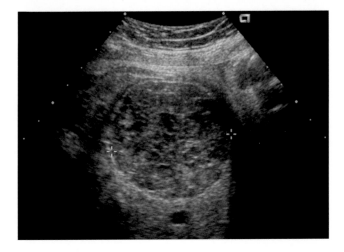

Case 74 Prenatal Left Ovarian Cyst/Torsion

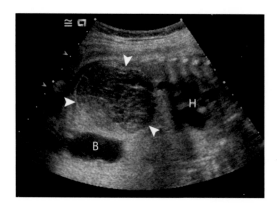
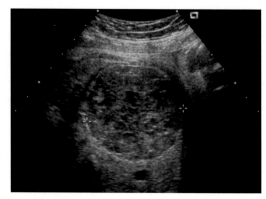

Findings

▶ Transabdominal sagittal image (left) and endovaginal transverse image (right) of the fetus reveal a complex cyst in the abdomen and pelvis (arrowheads). H indicates the heart and B indicates the bladder.

Differential diagnosis

The differential diagnosis consists of congenital cystic lesions, including enteric duplication cyst, lymphangioma or lymphatic malformation, and mature cystic teratoma. Gut signature in the wall suggests duplication, irregular borders and multilocular appearance suggest lymphangioma, and the finding of calcifications or fat suggests mature teratoma.

Teaching points

▶ Newborn infant girls may have ovarian cysts due to the influence of maternal hormones. These may be very large and predispose the ovary to torsion.
▶ Echogenic debris within the cyst suggests torsion.
▶ Although these are ovarian in origin, the pelvis of infants is small and the cyst commonly occupies much of the abdomen.
▶ May present as palpable midline abdominal mass on initial physical exam.

Next steps in management

Treatment for large cysts is laparoscopic surgery or percutaneous aspiration. Smaller cysts may be followed.

Further reading

1. Ratani RS, Cohen HL, Fiore E. Pediatric gynecologic ultrasound. Ultrasound Q. 2004 Sep;20(3):127–139.
2. Garel L, Dubois J, Grignon A, et al. US of the pediatric female pelvis: a clinical perspective. Radiographics. 2001 Nov–Dec; 21(6):1393–1407

Part 4   Spine

History

▶ 14-year-old boy with scapular deformity and limited range of motion of left shoulder.

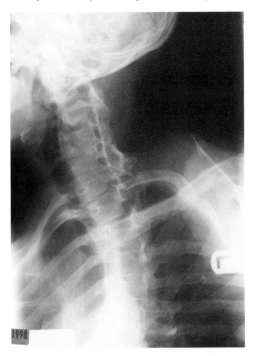

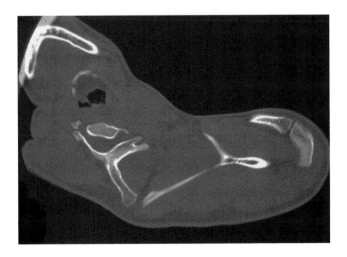

Case 75   Klippel-Feil Anomaly with Sprengel Deformity

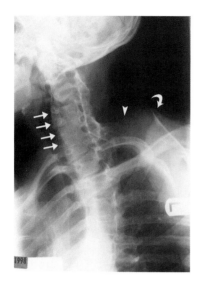
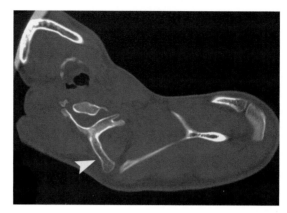

Findings

▶ Oblique radiograph of the cervical spine (left) shows fusion of the lower four cervical vertebral bodies (arrows) and the T1 vertebral body. Abnormal position of the scapula (curved arrow) is due to the bony bridge between the spine and the scapula, or omovertebral bone (arrowhead).

▶ The omovertebral bone (arrowhead), bridging the posterior elements of the vertebral body to the medial scapula, is better depicted on the CT image (right).

Differential diagnosis

Vertebral body fusion alone may be due to juvenile idiopathic arthritis.

Teaching points

▶ The Klippel-Feil anomaly consists of fusion of cervical vertebral bodies, which is actually due to a failure of segmentation. Patients often have short neck, low posterior hairline, and decreased range of neck motion.

▶ Frequently associated with the Klippel-Feil anomaly is the Sprengel deformity of abnormally rotated scapula due to the presence of the omovertebral bone shown above.

▶ Other associated spinal anomalies include occipitalization of the atlas, basilar impression, anomalies of the dens, and scoliosis.

▶ Associated neurologic abnormalities should be sought and may include Chiari I malformation, syringohydromyelia, diastematomyelia, and neurenteric cyst.

▶ Associated anomalies of other organ systems include genitourinary, cardiac, ear, and limb anomalies.

Next steps in management

CT and MR well demonstrate the full spectrum of the spinal malformation and associated neurologic abnormalities. Surgery may be required for neurologic complications.

Further reading

1. Klimo P, Rao G, Brockmeyer D. Congenital anomalies of the cervical spine. Neurosurg Clin North Am. 2007 Jul:18(3): 463–478.
2. Samartzis D, Herman J, Lubicky JP, Shen FH. Sprengel's deformity in Klippel-Feil syndrome. Spine. 2007 Aug 15; 32(18):E512–E516.

History

▶ 6-year-old with spine deformity.

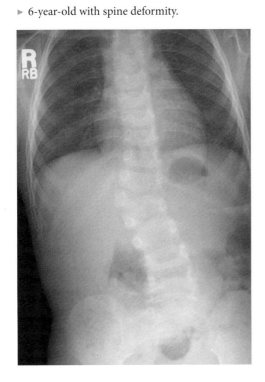

Case 76 Congenital Scoliosis due to Hemivertebra

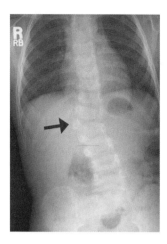

Findings

▶ L1 is a hemivertebra with only the right pedicle present (arrow). This deformity causes acute convex right scoliosis.

Differential diagnosis

Scoliosis is frequently idiopathic. The most common form is the adolescent type, which develops after 10 years of age, usually in girls. The primary curve is convex right thoracic or thoracolumbar and the secondary curve is convex left lumbar, forming an S configuration. Idiopathic scoliosis may also occur in infants. Atypical clinical or radiographic features such as rapid progression, pain, erosion of pedicles, or widening of neural foramina or evidence of dysraphism should prompt further evaluation with MRI. Painful scoliosis may be caused by osteoid osteoma of the spine. Patients with severe neuromuscular disorders often develop gentle C-shaped curvature of the spine.

Teaching points

▶ Congenital spine deformities may result from abnormalities of formation or segmentation. Examples of the former include hemivertebra, butterfly vertebra, or wedge vertebra. Examples of the latter include block vertebra.

▶ Associated abnormalities of the spinal cord such as syringohydromyelia, cord tethering, and diastematomyelia are seen in up to 20%, and MR imaging of the spine is indicated in congenital kyphoscoliosis.

▶ Patients with vertebral anomalies also have an increased incidence of rib anomalies (fused or bifid ribs) as well as cardiac and renal anomalies. Vertebral anomalies, particularly hemi- and butterfly vertebra, are part of the VACTERL association.

Next steps in management

Surgical resection of the hemivertebra and spinal fusion correct the cosmetic deformity and prevent progression of neurologic sequelae. If present, associated tethered cord is released and syrinx drained.

Further reading

1. Durand DJ, Huisman TA, Carrino JA. MR imaging features of common variant spinal anatomy. Magn Reson Imag Clin North Am. 2010 Nov;18(4):717–726.
2. Malfair D, Flemming AK, Dvorak MF, et al. Radiographic evaluation of scoliosis: review. AJR Am J Roentgenol. 2010 Mar;194(3 Suppl):S8–S22.

History

▶ 8-month-old girl with recurrent UTI and constipation.

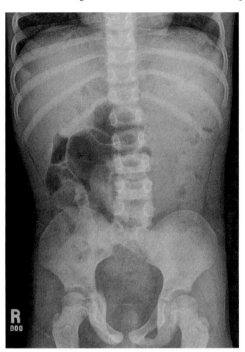

Case 77 Caudal Regression Syndrome (CRS)

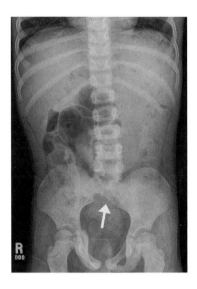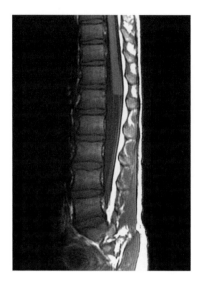

Findings

- ► AP radiograph (left) shows absence of the sacrum and lower lumbar spine (arrow).
- ► Sagittal T1-weighted MR in an older patient (right) shows a high wedge-shaped conus medullaris (arrowhead).

Differential diagnosis

Differential includes other spinal anomalies.

Teaching points

- ► Maldevelopment of the caudal cell mass causes a range of anomalies, including CRS, terminal myelocystocele, tethered cord syndrome (tight filum terminale), anterior sacral meningocele, and sacrococcygeal teratoma.
- ► Caudal regression consists of a wide spectrum of abnormalities ranging from sacral agenesis to sirenomelia (fused lower extremity). Up to 20% of affected patients are infants of diabetic mothers.
- ► CRS is associated with other anomalies of the spine and cord and GI and GU tracts, including spinal segmentation anomalies, dysraphism, split cord malformation, neurogenic bladder, anorectal malformation, VACTERL association, and the Currarino triad (sacral anomaly, anorectal malformation, and presacral teratoma or anterior meningocele).
- ► Two types
  - ▪ Type I—more severe; high blunted or wedge-shaped conus medullaris
  - ▪ Type II—less severe; low, tethered cord

Next steps in management

MRI is indicated to demonstrate associated anomalies of the spinal cord.

Further reading

1. Barkovich AJ. Congenital anomalies of the spine. In: Pediatric Neuroimaging. Philadelphia: Lippincott, Williams, & Wilkins; 2005:735–744.
2. Tortori-Donati P, Rossi A, Cama A. Spinal dysraphism: a review of neuroradiological features with embryological correlations and proposal for a new classification. Neuroradiology. 2000;42:471–491.

Part 5 **Neuroradiology**

History

► 1-week-old 28-week premature infant.

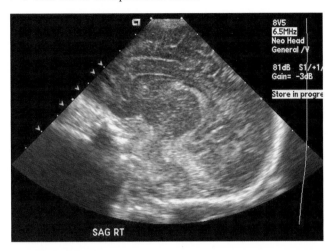

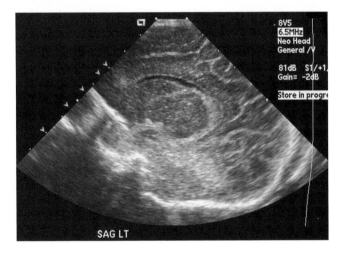

Case 78   Right Germinal Matrix Hemorrhage (GMH)

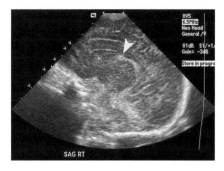 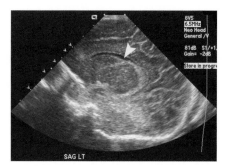

Findings

▶ Sagittal US image of the right caudothalamic groove (left) shows an echogenic rounded hemorrhage (arrowhead) immediately anterior to the curve of the echogenic choroid plexus of the lateral ventricle.

▶ Comparison sagittal US of the left side shows the normal appearance of the caudothalamic groove (arrowhead).

Differential diagnosis

The normal choroid plexus is echogenic but symmetric, so asymmetry suggests hemorrhage. Acute hemorrhage is isoechoic to choroid plexus. In the lateral ventricle, acute hemorrhage may be juxtaposed to the choroid plexus and go unrecognized. If the echogenic material layers in the occipital horn of the lateral ventricle, it is hemorrhage rather than choroid plexus.

Teaching points

▶ The risk of neonatal intracranial hemorrhage increases with decreasing gestational age. The germinal matrix is a highly vascular region of neuronal precursor cells that is prone to hemorrhage in stressed neonates with deficient autoregulation of cerebral blood flow.

▶ The Papile grading system of intracranial hemorrhage is still used, but many authors now prefer to use descriptive terms for several reasons. Not all ventricular dilation is due to intraventricular hemorrhage (IVH). Also, it is now recognized that intraparenchymal hemorrhage is not due to rupture of IVH through the ventricular wall but rather a hemorrhagic venous infarct due to decreased flow in the periventricular terminal veins.

  ■ Grade I = GMH without IVH
  ■ Grade II = IVH without ventricular dilation
  ■ Grade III = IVH with ventricular dilation
  ■ Grade IV = Intraparenchymal hemorrhage

▶ As the hemorrhage evolves, it becomes smaller and more hypoechoic or even cystic.

Next steps in management

Screening ultrasound is performed in asymptomatic neonates born at less than 32 weeks gestational age at 4 to 7 days of age. If hemorrhage is discovered, follow-up ultrasound is performed.

Further reading

1. Argyropoulou MI. Brain lesions in preterm infants: initial diagnosis and follow-up. Pediatr Radiol. 2010 Jun;40(6):811–818.
2. Taylor GA. New concepts in the pathogenesis of germinal matrix and intraparenchymal hemorrhage in premature infants. AJNR Am J Neuroradiol. 1997;18:231–232.

History

▶ 2-month-old with midline hemangioma in lumbosacral region.

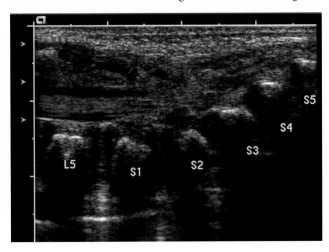

Case 79   Closed Dysraphism with Lipomyelocele and Tethering

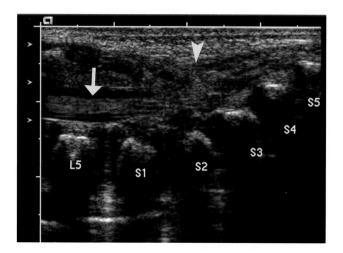
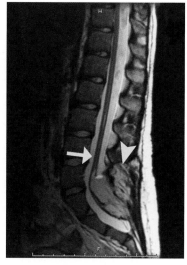

Findings

▶ Sagittal ultrasound of the spine (left) shows straight extension of the cauda equina (arrow) past S1 into an echogenic mass (arrowhead).

▶ Sagittal T2-weighted MR in an older patient (right) shows lack of tapering of the spinal cord and nerve roots (arrow) extending into a fatty mass that protrudes through the posterior spinal elements (arrowhead).

Differential diagnosis

Differential includes other spinal anomalies.

Teaching points

▶ Failure of proper closure of the neuropore and separation of the neural elements from adjacent mesenchyme or ectoderm gives rise to a variety of abnormalities of the spine, including open and closed spinal dysraphism, dorsal dermal sinus, and intracanal lipomas.

▶ Spinal ultrasound can be performed up to age 6 months. The level of the conus is determined by counting from the last rib at T12 or from the lower sacrum or coccyx. If the lowest ossification center is rounded, it is C1. If it is at all squared, it is S5. The conus should be no lower than the pedicles of L2. Other findings suggesting tethering of the cord include lack of tapering of the conus, lack of normal movement of caudal nerve roots due to CSF pulsations, and nerve roots in nondependent position in the dorsal spinal canal when the child is prone. Spinal dysraphism is best seen on axial images. Other findings that should be sought are a dorsal dermal sinus from the dimple, best seen in the sagittal plane. Also, dermoids or epidermoids of the tract and meningoceles should be sought.

▶ On MR imaging, sagittal and axial T1-weighted images are best to show fat in the spinal canal and in the filum.

Next steps in management

Surgical repair is indicated.

Further reading

1. Barkovich AJ. Congenital anomalies of the spine. In: Pediatric Neuroimaging. Philadelphia: Lippincott, Williams, & Wilkins; 2005:704–735.
2. Tortori-Donati P, Rossi A, Cama A. Spinal dysraphism: a review of neuroradiological features with embryological correlations and proposal for a new classification. Neuroradiology. 2000;42:471–491.

History

▶ 3-month-old with enlarging head circumference.

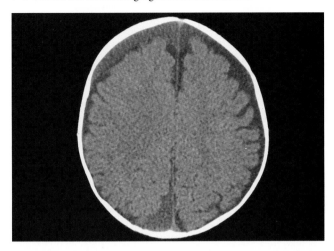

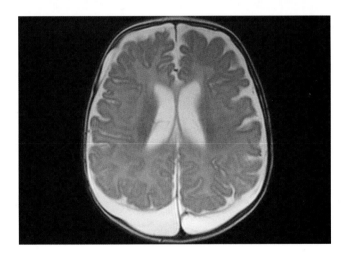

Case 80 Bilateral Subdural Hematomas due to Inflicted Trauma

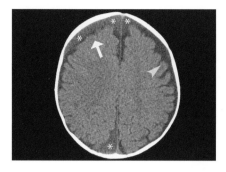 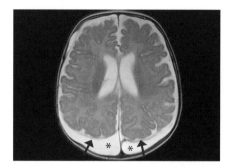

Findings

▶ Initial CT image (right) shows dense extraxial fluid (asterisks). On the right side, the gyri are compressed (arrow), while on the left, where the fluid is not dense, the gyri are not compressed (arrowhead). Most of the fluid on the left side is subarachnoid fluid, while the dense material causing gyral compression on the right is subdural hemorrhage.

▶ Axial T2-weighted MR image at a lower level shows hyperintense fluid posterior to the brain in a supine patient (asterisks). Note the vessels compressed against the brain (arrows). This is subdural fluid.

Differential diagnosis

Subdural fluid must be distinguished from benign expanded subarachnoid spaces. If the fluid does not follow the appearance of CSF in the ventricles, then it represents hematoma or infected fluid.

Teaching points

▶ Subdural hematomas result from shear forces and are much more common in inflicted trauma than in accidental trauma. Interhemispheric subdural hematomas are particularly suspicious.

▶ It was previously thought that subdurals of different signal intensity were definitely of different ages, but this finding can occur in a single traumatic episode, as an arachnoid tear may occur, allowing CSF to mix with blood on one side and not the other.

▶ Cerebral edema is the most common imaging finding in inflicted trauma but is nonspecific. In severe cases, the cerebrum may be diffusely hypoattenuating due to edema, while the attenuation of the cerebellum and deep gray nuclei is preserved (white cerebellum sign).

▶ Skull fractures are also common in accidental trauma. Features that suggest inflicted trauma include stellate configuration, depression, diastasis, or bilateral findings.

▶ MR or CT venography is helpful to exclude venous sinus thrombosis as a cause of cerebral hemorrhage.

Next steps in management

Child Protective Services must be notified right away. Skeletal survey should be performed.

Further reading

1. Fernando S, Obaldo RE, Walsh IR, Lowe LH. Neuroimaging of nonaccidental head trauma: pitfalls and controversies. Pediatr Radiol. 2008;38:827–838
2. Poussaint TY, Moeller KK. Imaging of pediatric head trauma. Neuroimaging Clin North Am 2002;12:271–294, ix.

History

▶ 1-week-old ex-28-week premature baby boy (first image). Second image is 8 weeks later.

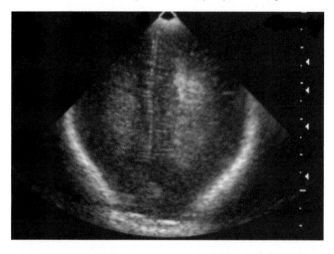

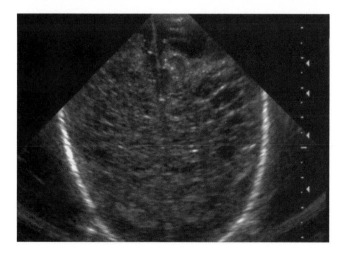

Case 81 Periventricular Leukomalacia

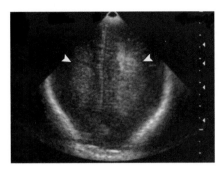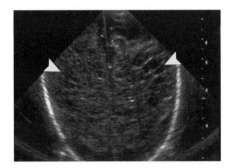

Findings

▶ Coronal US image obtained acutely (left) shows increased echogenicity in the white matter posterior to the atria of the lateral ventricles (arrowheads), left greater than right.

▶ Delayed coronal US image of posterior parietal lobes (right) shows cystic changes in the periventricular white matter (arrowheads), left greater than right.

Differential diagnosis

The white matter in the periatrial regions is normally somewhat echogenic but should be symmetric and no more echogenic than the choroid plexus. Paraventricular parenchymal hemorrhage is usually unilateral, fan-shaped and pointing toward the ventricle, and associated with intraventricular hemorrhage.

Teaching points

▶ Ischemia and hypoxia and immature autoregulation of cerebral blood flow lead to infarcts in the watershed zones, which in the premature brain is the periventricular white matter.

▶ Initial ultrasound findings show bilateral increased echogenicity of the periventricular white matter in the periatrial regions without mass effect. Frontal white matter near the foramen of Monro may also be affected. On delayed imaging coalescent small cysts develop in these areas.

▶ Delayed MR imaging shows thinning of the periventricular white matter posteriorly more than anteriorly, dilation of the lateral ventricles with irregular margins, T2-hyperintensity within remaining white matter representing gliosis, and thinning of the posterior corpus callosum. In severe cases, gray matter injury may also be apparent affecting the cortex, thalami, and deep gray nuclei.

Next steps in management

If echogenic white matter is detected on ultrasound, follow-up ultrasound will show cystic changes developing in the affected areas in 1 to 3 weeks. Delayed MR can help to show the anatomic sequelae and help to predict functional outcome.

Further reading

1. Bulas DI, Vezina GL. Preterm axonic injury. Radiologic evaluation. Radiol Clin North Am. 1999 Nov;37(6):1147–1161.
2. Argyropoulou MI. Brain lesions in preterm infants: initial diagnosis and follow-up. Pediatr Radiol. 2010 Jun;40(6):811–818.

History

▶ 6-year-old with headache and altered mental status.

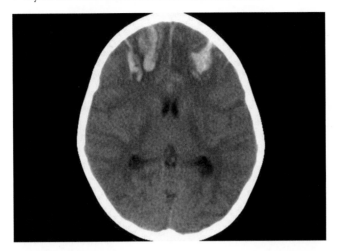

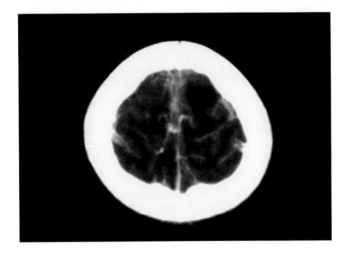

Case 82 Superior Sagittal Sinus Thrombosis with Hemorrhagic Venous Infarcts

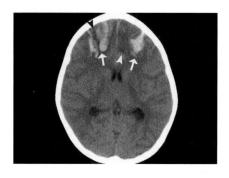 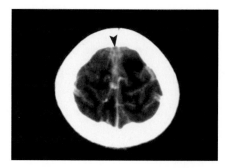

Findings

▶ Unenhanced axial CT image (left) shows bilateral foci of hyperattenuating acute parenchymal hemorrhage (arrows) and hypoattenuating edema (arrowheads) in a parasagittal distribution.

▶ Axial CT venogram image demonstrates a filling defect in the superior sagittal sinus (arrowhead).

Differential diagnosis

Normal structures that may be mistaken for venous sinus thrombosis include arachnoid granulations, which are well defined and focal, and normal asymmetry of flow in the transverse and sigmoid sinuses.

Teaching points

▶ Cerebral sinovenous thrombosis is caused by trauma (birth, head injury), infection (meningitis, adjacent paranasal sinus infection), severe dehydration, and hypercoagulable states. The most common sites are the superior sagittal sinus (SSS), straight sinus, and transverse sinus.

▶ On unenhanced CT images, the thrombosed dural venous sinus appears abnormally dense. With contrast enhancement, the surrounding dura enhances, but the thrombus does not. In the SSS, this finding is called the "empty delta" sign.

▶ MR imaging may show lack of the normal flow void on T1- or T2-weighted images and lack of the normal flow artifact in the phase-encoding direction. The appearance on MR is affected by the evolution of blood products. MR venography can be performed with 2D time-of-flight (TOF) or 2D phase-contrast imaging. Subacute hemorrhage may be hyperintense on T1 and will not show as a defect on TOF sequences. Both types of sequences can be adversely affected by properties of flow such as slow flow or in-plane flow. 3D post-contrast venography is not affected by these artifacts.

▶ On CT venous infarcts are low in attenuation due to vasogenic edema. Subcortical hemorrhage is frequent.

Next steps in management

Treatment is systemic anticoagulation and therapy for the underlying cause.

Further reading

1. Jonas Kimchi T, Lee SK, Agid R, et al. Cerebral sinovenous thrombosis in children. Neuroimaging Clin North Am. 2007 May;17(2):239–244
2. Rodallec MH, Krainik A, Feydy A, et al. Cerebral venous thrombosis and multidetector CT angiography: tips and tricks. Radiographics. 2006 Oct;26 Suppl 1:S5–S18.

History

► 8-year-old boy with developmental delay.

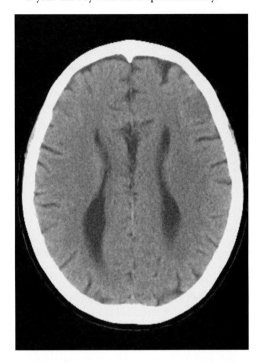

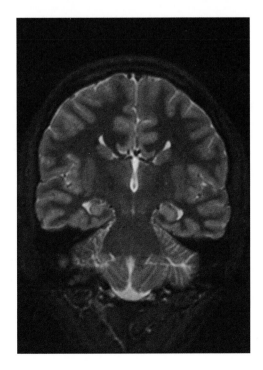

Case 83 Agenesis of the Corpus Callosum

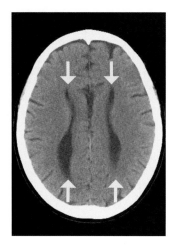
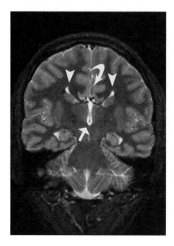

Findings

▶ Axial CT image shows an abnormally straight orientation of the lateral ventricles resembling racing car tires (arrows). No white matter is seen crossing the midline.

▶ Coronal T2-weighted MR image reveals a high-riding third ventricle (arrow) and lack of white matter tracks crossing the midline (curved arrow). The sagittally oriented tracks (Probst bundles) cause lateral deviation of the frontal horns (arrowheads) so that they resemble steer horns.

Differential diagnosis

The differential includes dysgenesis of the corpus callosum, which shows incomplete but similar findings.

Teaching points

▶ The corpus callosum generally forms from front to back (except the rostrum, which forms last). In agenesis, no corpus callosum is seen. In dysgenesis, the posterior portions and the rostrum are absent.

▶ In the absence of formation of the corpus callosum, white matter fibers do not cross the midline, but instead run parallel to the falx on either side. The presence of these fibers in this position (Probst bundles) deforms the frontal horns of the lateral ventricles so that they are crescent-shaped in the coronal plane. The third ventricle is elevated and slightly widened. The orientation of the lateral ventricles is more parallel than normal. The frontal horns are much smaller than the posterior lateral ventricles and, in their parallel orientation, resemble the tires of a racing car.

▶ Associated anomalies include:
  ▪ Colpocephaly—enlargement of atria and occipital horns of the lateral ventricles
  ▪ Interhemispheric cyst or lipoma
  ▪ Chiari II malformation
  ▪ Dandy-Walker malformation
  ▪ Cephalocele
  ▪ Heterotopic gray matter

Next steps in management

Associated malformations should be sought on MRI.

Further reading

1. Barkovich AJ. Magnetic resonance imaging: role in the understanding of cerebral malformations. Brain Dev. 2002 Jan;24(1):2–12.
2. Wright LB, James CA, Glasier CM. Congenital cerebral and cerebrovascular anomalies: magnetic resonance imaging. Top Magn Reson Imaging. 2001 Dec;12(6):361–374.

History

▶ 8-year-old boy with developmental delay.

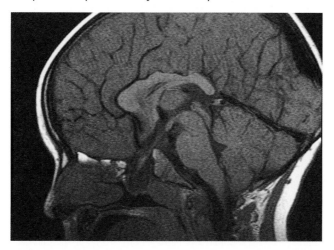

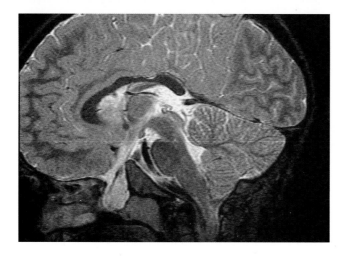

Case 84 Transsphenoidal Cephalocele

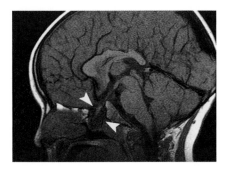 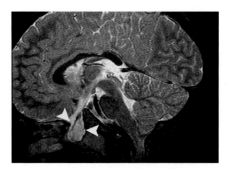

Findings

▶ Sagittal T1- (left) and T2-weighted (right) images show herniation of meninges, cerebrospinal fluid, and the optic chiasm (arrowheads) through a defect in the sphenoid bone into the posterior nasopharynx.

Differential diagnosis

The differential diagnostic considerations for frontoethmoidal and nasal lesions include nasal glial heterotopias (herniated glial tissue without communication with the intracranial contents) and dermoids/epidermoids.

Teaching points

▶ A cephalocele is the herniation of intracranial contents through a defect in the skull. A meningocele is a subtype of cephalocele in which the herniated material consists of only meninges and CSF. An encephalocele or meningoencephalocele is a subtype in which brain tissue is also herniated.

▶ The most common site for cephaloceles in the Western Hemisphere is the occipital region, usually in girls, while the most common site in Southeast Asia is the frontoethmoidal region, predominantly in boys.

▶ Large cephaloceles may contain large portions of brain tissue, ventricles, and dural venous sinuses. Elongated ventricles may point to the defect. Smaller cephaloceles may contain disorganized neural tissue.

▶ CT is superior for demonstrating the bony defect, which may be helpful in small nasofrontal lesions. MR better demonstrates involved neural and vascular structures as well as associated intracranial anomalies, such as dysgenesis of the corpus callosum, absence of the septum pellucidum, neuronal migration anomalies, and Dandy-Walker malformation.

▶ Skull base cephaloceles tend to occur at sutures. Anterior herniations are called sincipital cephaloceles, which always have an external mass in the midline or in the orbit. Basal cephaloceles are anterior and middle skull base cephaloceles without external masses, and include transsphenoidal cephaloceles. Intracranial contents may extend into the nasopharynx.

Next steps in management

Preoperative MRA is important for mapping the involved arteries and venous sinuses.

Further reading

1. Connor SE. Imaging of skull base cephaloceles and cerebrospinal fluid leaks. Clin Radiol. 2010 Oct;65:832–841.
2. Hedlund G. Congenital frontonasal masses: developmental anatomy, malformations, and MR imaging. Pediatr Radiol. 2006 Jul;36(7):647–662.

History

▶ 19-month-old boy with developmental delay.

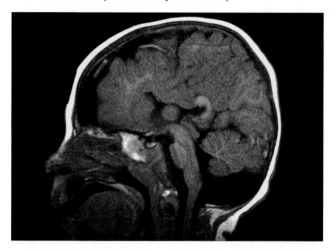

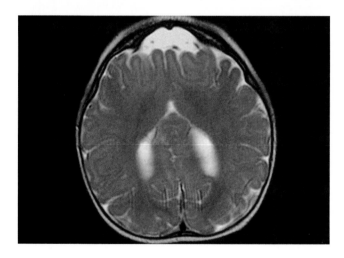

Case 85   Semilobar Holoprosencephaly

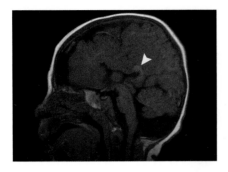 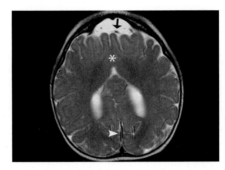

Findings

▶ Sagittal T1-weighted MR image (left) demonstrates only the splenium of the corpus callosum (arrowhead).

▶ Axial T2-weighted image (right) shows only the posterior falx (arrowhead). There is posterior separation into lateral ventricles but no frontal horns. The frontal lobes are fused (asterisk). A single (azygos) anterior cerebral artery is seen (arrow).

Differential diagnosis

The presence of only the posterior portion of the corpus callosum occurs only in the holoprosencephaly spectrum as the corpus callosum forms from front to back. In dysgenesis of the corpus callosum, only the anterior genu and anterior body are present.

Teaching points

▶ The holoprosencephaly spectrum is caused by lack of complete separation of the prosencephalon into two cerebral hemispheres. Absence of the septum pellucidum is a constant finding in this diverse spectrum of abnormalities.

▶ In alobar holoprosencephaly, the most severe form, there is complete failure of separation and absence of all midline structures—septum pellucidum, corpus callosum, falx, and interhemispheric fissure. There is a single monoventricle with a crescent of fused brain anteriorly. The monoventricle communicates with a large dorsal cyst and the thalami and basal ganglia are fused. A single azygos anterior cerebral artery may be noted. Facial anomalies are common and include hypotelorism or cyclopia, single nostril, proboscis, and cleft lip and palate.

▶ Semilobar holoprosencephaly describes partial separation that proceeds posterior to anterior. The midline structures are formed posteriorly but absent anteriorly. Facial anomalies are mild.

▶ Lobar holoprosencephaly is the mildest form, with absence of the septum pellucidum and small frontal horns of the lateral ventricles. The differential diagnostic consideration is septo-optic dysplasia with absence of the septum pellucidum and hypoplasia of the optic nerves and chiasm. Patients may have normal intelligence.

Next steps in management

MR imaging best shows the spectrum of anomalies.

Further reading

1. Barkovich AJ. Magnetic resonance imaging: role in the understanding of cerebral malformations. Brain Dev. 2002 Jan;24(1):2–12.
2. Wright LB, James CA, Glasier CM. Congenital cerebral and cerebrovascular anomalies: magnetic resonance imaging. Top Magn Reson Imaging. 2001 Dec;12(6):361–374.

History

▶ 2-year-old with developmental delay.

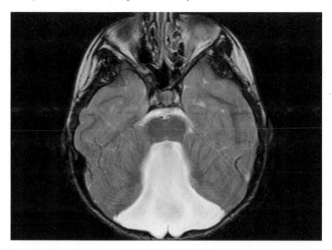

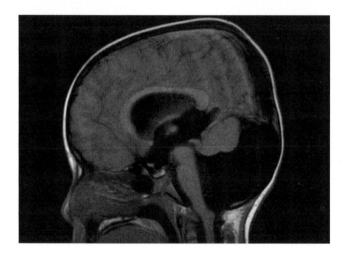

Case 86　Dandy-Walker Malformation

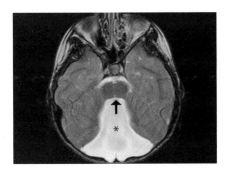 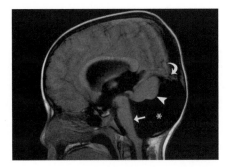

Findings

▶ Axial (left) and sagittal (right) MR images reveal enlargement of the posterior fossa, which is filled with a large cyst (*) that freely communicates with the fourth ventricle and elevates the tentorium cerebelli (curved arrow) and compresses the brainstem anteriorly (arrow). The cerebellar hemispheres are widely separated and the cerebellar vermis (arrowhead) is hypoplastic.

Differential diagnosis

The differential includes other entities of the Dandy-Walker complex, posterior fossa arachnoid cyst, and Blake's pouch cyst (herniation of the inferior portion of the fourth ventricle through the foramen of Magendie). These are best differentiated by evaluating the cerebellar vermis, which is hypoplastic or absent in Dandy-Walker malformation.

Teaching points

▶ Dandy-Walker malformation is now considered part of a continuum of developmental posterior fossa cysts. The classic malformation consists of the findings above. The term "Dandy-Walker variant" is the subject of some debate as to whether it represents a distinct entity. The term is generally applied to the finding of mild inferior vermian hypoplasia without enlargement of the posterior fossa. "Mega cisterna magna" describes an enlarged cisterna magna with normal cerebellar vermis.

▶ The neurologic outcome is determined by the associated hydrocephalus and supratentorial anomalies, including dysgenesis of the corpus callosum, gray matter heterotopias, cortical malformations, holoprosencephaly, and cephaloceles.

Next steps in management

MR imaging best shows the findings of Dandy-Walker malformation and the associated supratentorial anomalies. Sagittal images best show the cerebellar vermis. Treatment consists of shunting the posterior fossa cyst and, if necessary, the lateral ventricles.

Further reading

1. Patel S, Barkovich A. Analysis and classification of cerebellar malformations. AJNR Am J Neuroradiol. 2002;23:1074–1087.
2. Barkovich AJ, Kjos BO, Norman D, Edwards MSB. Revised classification of posterior fossa cysts and cyst-like malformations based on results of multiplanar MR imaging. AJNR Am J Neuroradiol. 1997;18:231–232.

History

▶ 6-year-old with known diagnosis.

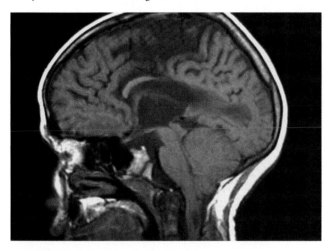

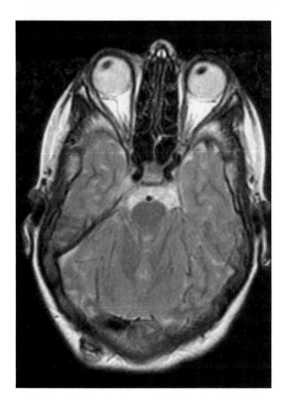

Case 87 Chiari II Malformation

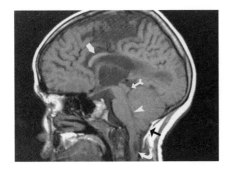 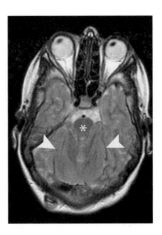

Findings

- ▶ Sagittal T1-weighted MR image (left) shows a small posterior fossa with herniation of the cerebellar vermis (arrow) through the foramen magnum, near obliteration of the fourth ventricle (arrowhead), and beaking of the tectum (tailed arrow). Additional findings include a cervical cord syrinx (curved arrow) and dysgenesis of the corpus callosum (block arrow) with absence of the splenium, posterior body, and rostrum.
- ▶ Axial T2-weighted MR image (right) shows heart-shaped towering cerebellum herniating through the tentorium (arrowheads) and narrowing the tectum (*).

Differential diagnosis

The above findings in concert are specific for Chiari II malformation. Ectopia of the cerebellar tonsils with a beaked appearance and the cord syrinx without the other findings would constitute Chiari I malformation.

Teaching points

- ▶ Chiari II malformation consists of a constellation of abnormalities of the supra- and infratentorial brain and spine. Virtually all patients with Chiari II malformation have hydrocephalus and lumbosacral dysraphism with myelomeningocele.
- ▶ The posterior fossa is abnormally small and its contents are herniated through the tentorium cerebelli and the foramen magnum. Secondary deformities include "towering" configuration of the cerebellum, a beaked appearance of the tectum, absent or slit-like fourth ventricle, and a cervicomedullary kink where the cervical cord is fixed by the dentate ligaments.
- ▶ Supratentorial findings include hydrocephalus, large massa intermedia, dysgenesis of the corpus callosum, and fenestration of the falx cerebri with interdigitation of gyri across the midline.
- ▶ Prior to age 6 months, there are increased convolutional markings in the skull ("lacunar" skull), which is thought to represent a mesodermal defect rather than the result of hydrocephalus.

Next steps in management

The myelomeningocele is closed and a ventricular shunt is placed at birth. Patients are monitored for shunt complications with low-dose CT as clinically indicated.

Further reading

1. Wolpert SM, Anderson M, Scott RM, et al. The Chiari II malformation: MR imaging evaluation. AJNR Am J Neuroradiol. 1987;8:783–791.
2. Naidich TP, McLone DG, Fulling KH. The Chiari II malformation: Part IV. The hindbrain deformity. Neuroradiology. 1983;25(4):179–197.

History

► 4-year-old boy with seizures.

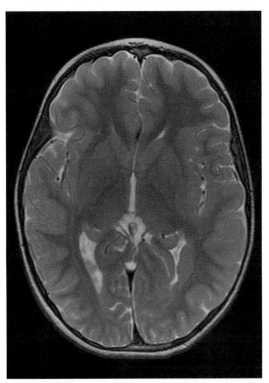

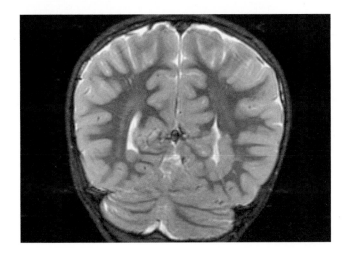

Case 88   Subependymal Heterotopic Gray Matter

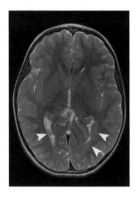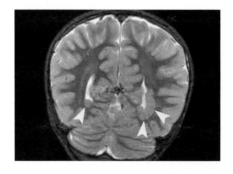

Findings

▶ Axial (left) and coronal (right) T2-weighted MR images demonstrate large areas of material of the same appearance as gray matter along the margins of the atria of the lateral ventricles (arrowheads).

Differential diagnosis

The subependymal nodules of tuberous sclerosis occur in the same location, but heterotopic gray matter always follows the signal of gray matter while nodules of tuberous sclerosis vary in signal depending on whether or not they are calcified.

Teaching points

▶ Neuronal migration anomalies represent a spectrum of arrest of normal migration of neurons from the subependymal regions to the surface of the brain. Patients usually present with seizures, less commonly with developmental delay.

▶ In lissencephaly, the most severe form, the brain is smooth with thick cortex without gyri. The brain has a "figure-of-8" configuration.

▶ Other forms include pachygyria and polymicrogyria (PMG), which appear similar on imaging. The cortex appears thickened and irregular. PMG is associated with congenital cytomegalovirus, Aicardi syndrome, and chromosomal anomalies. Anomalies of cortical venous drainage are often noted.

▶ Hemimegalencephaly is a hamartomatous overgrowth of all or a portion of a cerebral hemisphere due to defects in all phases of cortical development. The ipsilateral lateral ventricle is often enlarged.

▶ Gray matter heterotopias are usually nodular foci that may occur anywhere from the ependymal surface to just below the normal gray matter.

▶ Band heterotopia is a continuous line of gray matter in the subcortical white matter. This condition is found only in girls.

▶ Schizencephaly is a migrational anomaly in which there is a gray matter-lined cleft (see Case 91, De Morsier syndrome).

Next steps in management

MRI is best for demonstrating these abnormalities and associated anomalies. Surface coils may be helpful if EEG localizes to a specific location.

Further reading

1. Abdel Razek AA, Kandell AY, Elsorogy LG, Elmongy A, Basett AA. Disorders of cortical formation: MR imaging features. AJNR Am J Neuroradiol. 2009 Jan;30(1):4–11.
2. Barkovich AJ, Raybaud CA. Neuroimaging in disorders of cortical development. Neuroimaging Clin North Am 2004;14:231–254, vii.

History

► 3-month-old with abnormally shaped head.

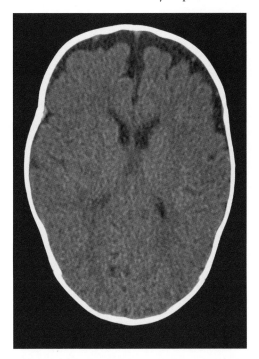

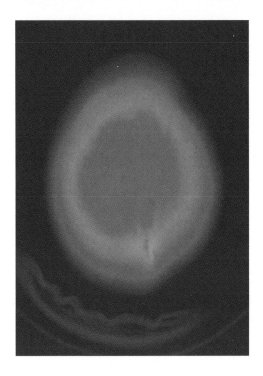

Case 89 Craniosynostosis—Sagittal Suture

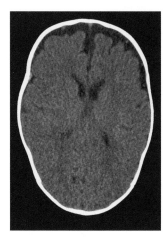
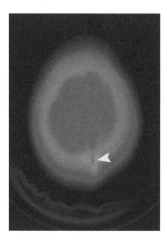

Findings

▶ Axial CT image shows an abnormally elongated skull shape in the anterior-posterior plane with widest portion in the temporal region rather than the parietal region as in the normal skull—scaphocephaly.

▶ Axial CT image near vertex in bone window demonstrates absence of the normal lucent sagittal suture and linear sclerosis, or ridging, along its expected course (arrowhead).

Differential diagnosis

Positional deformation of the skull may result from the infant sleeping on its back (plagicephaly) or with head turned to the side while prone (NICU infants with pseudoscaphocephaly—widest part of skull is parietal region).

Teaching points

▶ Growth of the skull proceeds perpendicular to the long axis of the sutures. Synostosis of particular sutures causes specific abnormalities of the shape of the skull.
  ▪ Sagittal suture—scapho- or dolichocephaly
  ▪ Bilateral coronal sutures—brachicephaly—short, wide head
  ▪ Bilateral lambdoid sutures—turricephaly—upward growth
  ▪ Unilateral coronal or lambdoid—plagicephaly -- uplifted orbital roof ("harlequin eye") for coronal synostosis
  ▪ Metopic (normally closes by 3 months)—trigonocephaly—frontal beak above nose

▶ Most cases are sporadic but there is an association with syndromes involving mutations of fibroblast growth factor receptors, including Apert, Pfeiffer, and Crouzon syndromes and thanatophoric dysplasia, in which multiple sutures are frequently affected.

▶ Synostosis of all sutures may result in microcephaly. This condition may be associated with increased intracranial pressure or may occur secondary to decreased growth due to severe brain anomaly or injury.

▶ Evaluation for suspected craniosynostosis consists of a four-view skull series. Low-dose CT with 3D reconstructions helps in surgical planning.

Next steps in management

MR imaging detects associated brain anomalies and anomalous draining veins, which may affect the surgical approach. Surgical treatment is usually necessary as deformity is progressive and will affect brain development.

Further reading

1. Kirmi O, Lo SJ, Johnson D, Anslow P. Craniosynostosis: a radiological and surgical perspective. Semin Ultrasound CT MR. 2009 Dec;30(6):492–512.
2. Blaser SI. Abnormal skull shape. Pediatr Radiol. 2008 Jun;38 Suppl 3:S488–S496.

History

▶ 32-week fetus with abnormal ultrasound.

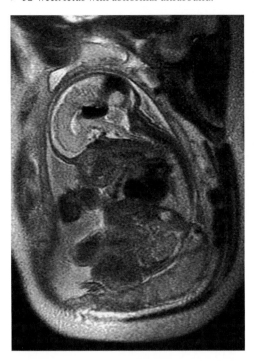

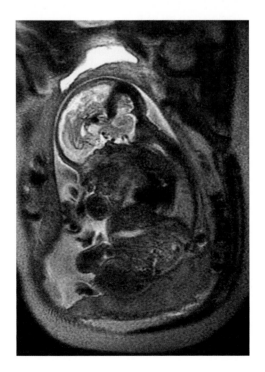

Case 90 Galenic Malformation

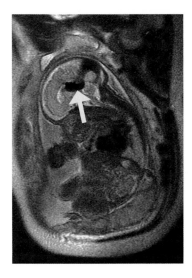 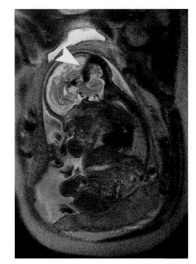

Findings

▶ Sagittal prenatal T2-weighted MR images show a large midline venous varix (arrow) draining into a persistent falcine sinus (arrowhead) and absence of the straight sinus.

Differential diagnosis

Differential includes two types of Galenic malformations.

Teaching points

▶ Galenic or vein of Galen malformations are anomalous connections between cerebral arteries and the vein of Galen or a primitive midline vein. Frequently, the straight sinus is absent and there is persistence of embryonic falcine and occipital sinuses, suggesting that the underlying cause may be in utero thrombosis of the straight sinus. There is a large midline varix, which represents persistence of the prosencephalic vein of Markowski.

▶ Cardiovascular anomalies are associated with Galenic malformations, particularly aortic coarctation and atrial septal defect.

▶ Two types:

  ▪ "Choroidal"—more than 90% of cases; these have multiple arteriovenous connections supplied by a large number of arteries causing massive AV shunting and intractable heart failure in the perinatal period.

  ▪ "Mural"—larger-caliber arteriovenous connections numbering four or fewer; patients are older and present with hydrocephalus, seizure, and/or hemorrhage.

▶ On imaging studies, high-velocity turbulent flow is observed in the midline varix. A large varix may cause hydrocephalus. Arteriovenous shunting may cause ischemic changes in the brain, which may be calcified at birth. The degree of ischemic or hemorrhagic damage has great prognostic import. Ischemic changes are better seen in unmyelinated white matter on T1-weighted images.

Next steps in management

Preferred therapy for both types is selective embolization, which has a high technical success rate.

Further reading

1. Wright LB, James CA, Glasier CM. Congenital cerebral and cerebrovascular anomalies: magnetic resonance imaging. Top Magn Reson Imaging. 2001 Dec;12(6):361–374.
2. Pearl M, Gomez J, Gregg L, Gailloud P. Endovascular management of vein of Galen aneurysmal malformations. Childs Nerv Syst. 2010 Oct;26(10):1367–1379.

History

▶ 2- year-old with blindness and developmental delay.

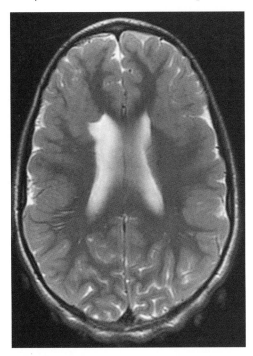

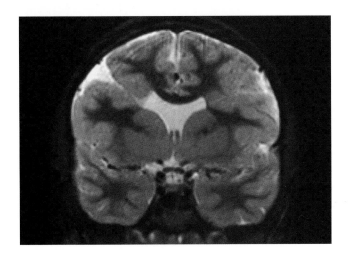

Case 91   Septo-optic Dysplasia with Schizencephaly—De Morsier Syndrome

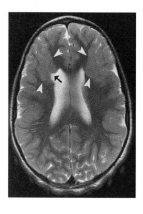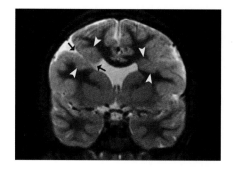

Findings

▶ Axial (left) and coronal (right) T2-weighted MR images show bilateral frontal gray matter-lined clefts (arrowheads). Note the outpouching of the right lateral ventricle wall extending toward the cleft and extension of the subarachnoid fluid on the outer surface of the cortex into the cleft on the right (arrows). The coronal image also shows absence of the septum pellucidum and a box-like configuration of the frontal horns of the lateral ventricles.

Differential diagnosis

Porencephalic cysts, which result from the destruction of gray and white matter, may mimic open-lip schizencephaly, but the cleft is lined by white matter.

Teaching points

▶ Schizencephaly is a cortical migrational anomaly in which gray matter-lined clefts communicating with the lateral ventricles are formed.

▶ In closed-lip schizencephaly, the gray matter-lined walls are apposed. In open-lip schizencephaly, there is a CSF-filled channel between the walls that extends from the lateral ventricle to the cortical surface.

▶ One third of patients have optic hypoplasia. Many also have absence of the septum pellucidum, and the septum pellucidum is almost always absent when the clefts involve both frontal lobes.

▶ Septo-optic dysplasia (De Morsier syndrome) is considered part of the holoprosencephaly spectrum and consists of absence or hypoplasia of the septum pellucidum and hypoplasia of the optic nerves. Two thirds of patients also have hypothalamic-pituitary dysfunction. Barkovich describes two distinct appearances. One group has partial absence of the septum pellucidum and schizencephaly and/or gray matter heterotopias. The other group demonstrates complete absence of the septum pellucidum and hypoplasia of cerebral white matter with ventriculomegaly.

Next steps in management

MR is superior to CT for demonstrating associated additional migrational anomalies and anomalous venous drainage.

Further reading

1. Scoffings DJ, Kurian KM. Congenital and acquired lesions of the septum pellucidum. Clin Radiol. 2008 Feb;63(2):210–219.
2. Abdel Razek AA, Kandell AY, Elsorogy LG, Elmongy A, Basett AA. Disorders of cortical formation: MR imaging features. AJNR Am J Neuroradiol. 2009 Jan;30(1):4–11.

History

► 5-week-old with absence of the left red reflex.

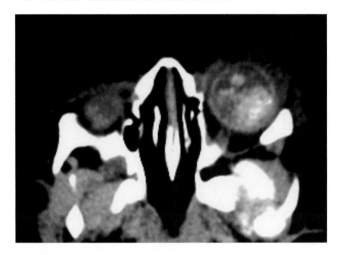

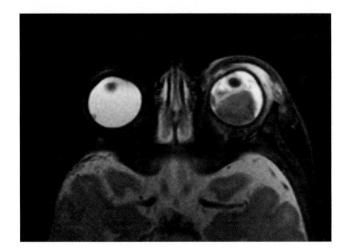

Case 92 Retinoblastoma

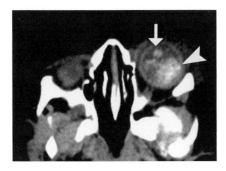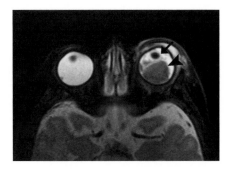

Findings

▸ Axial non-contrast CT of the orbits (left) shows a calcified mass (arrowhead) posterior to the lens (arrow).

▸ Axial T2-weighted MR image (right) shows the mass (arrowhead) is well defined and hypointense compared to vitreous. The arrow indicates the lens.

Differential diagnosis

The differential diagnosis of leukocoria (absence of red pupillary reflex) includes persistent hyperplastic primary vitreous (PHPV), Coats disease, and larval endophthalmitis due to Toxocara infection.

Teaching points

▸ Although rare, retinoblastoma is the most common tumor of the ocular globe in children. Retinoblastoma is an embryonal tumor.

▸ Heritable and nonheritable forms of retinoblastoma exist. The heritable form is a germline mutation that causes bilateral and multifocal tumors, with a younger peak age of incidence compared to the sporadic form. The mutation causes a loss of function of the tumor suppressor gene RB1. Histologically identical tumors may also arise in the pineal gland or parasellar region (trilateral retinoblastoma). Patients with RB1 germline mutations are also at increased risk of developing other tumors, including osteosarcoma, and the risk is increased if they are treated with external-beam radiation for bilateral ocular tumors.

▸ The most important distinguishing feature of retinoblastoma is calcification, so CT is the primary imaging modality in the evaluation of leukocoria. Ultrasound may also detect calcification but is not as sensitive for calcification as CT or for the evaluation of optic nerve or choroid invasion as CT or MR. MRI is superior to CT for the evaluation of intracranial spread of tumor. MRI should include dedicated images of the orbits as well as imaging of the entire brain. Post-gadolinium images should be fat-suppressed.

Next steps in management

Retinoblastoma is usually treated with enucleation.

Further reading

1. Chung EM, Specht CS, Schroeder JW. From the archives of the AFIP: pediatric orbit tumors and tumorlike lesions: neuroepithelial lesions of the ocular globe and optic nerve. Radiographics. 2007 Jul–Aug;27:1159–1186.
2. Vázquez E, Castellote A, Piqueras J, et al. Second malignancies in pediatric patients: imaging findings and differential diagnosis. Radiographics. 2003 Sep–Oct;23(5):1155–1172.

History

▸ 6-month-old with enlarging head circumference.

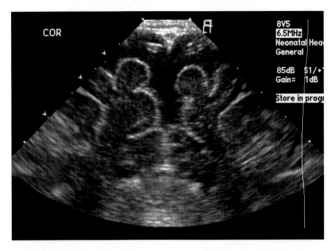

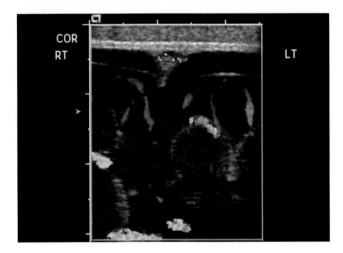

Case 93 Benign Expanded Subarachnoid Spaces

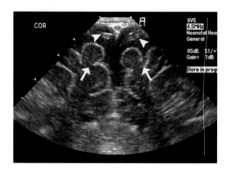 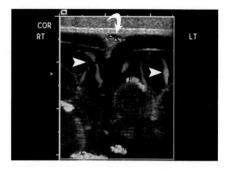

Findings

► Coronal ultrasound image through the anterior fontanelle (left) shows fluid with vessels traversing it (arrowheads). Note that the gyri are not compressed (arrows) and the fluid insinuates in between the gyri.

► Coronal color Doppler image (right) confirms vessels traversing the fluid (arrowheads). Curved arrow = superior sagittal sinus.

Differential diagnosis

Extra-axial fluid may occupy the subarachnoid or subdural spaces. There is normally a small amount of fluid in the subarachnoid spaces, but the subdural space is normally empty. The finding of subdural fluid is concerning for old hemorrhage due to inflicted or nonaccidental trauma. Cortical veins normally traverse the subarachnoid space to reach the superior sagittal sinus, so the finding of vessels traversing the fluid indicates that it is in the subarachnoid space. Also, the subarachnoid fluid does not compress the gyri. Additionally, normal subarachnoid fluid always follows the appearance of CSF in the ventricles on all imaging sequences and is found in the nondependent portion of the cranium. On the other hand, subdural fluid collections compress the gyri and the cortical veins against the surface of the brain so that the veins run parallel rather than perpendicular to the surface of the brain. Additionally, the subdural fluid collection may be loculated or separated by membranes.

Teaching points

► Benign expanded subarachnoid spaces has also been known as benign extra-axial fluid collections of infancy, benign subdural collections or effusion of infancy, or external hydrocephalus.

► Most patients present between 6 and 18 months of age with an enlarging head circumference and absence of neurologic signs. The condition resolves without sequelae.

Next steps in management

No further work-up or follow-up is required unless the patient develops neurologic signs or symptoms.

Further reading

1. Fernando S, Obaldo RE, Walsh IR, Lowe LH. Neuroimaging of nonaccidental head trauma: pitfalls and controversies. Pediatr Radiol. 2008;38:827–838
2. Carolan PL, McLaurin RL, Towbin RB, et al. Benign extracerebral fluid collections: a cause of macrocrania in infancy. Pediatr Neurosci. 1985–1986;12(3):140–144.

History

▶ 1-day-old with abnormal prenatal ultrasound in third trimester.

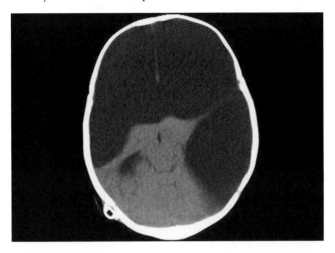

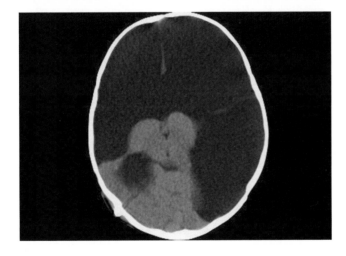

Case 94 Hydranencephaly

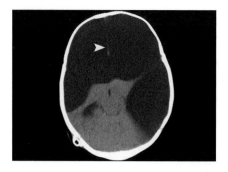 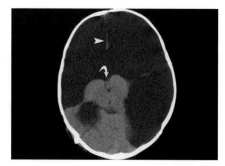

Findings

▶ Axial CT images of the brain reveal large, cystic spaces replacing the supratentorial brain with preservation of the brainstem and cerebellum. The finding of an anterior midline falx (arrowhead) excludes alobar holoprosencephaly. Further, midline structures are not fused (curved arrow).

Differential diagnosis

The differential diagnosis includes other conditions with large supratentorial cystic spaces—alobar holoprosencephaly and severe hydrocephalus. Alobar holoprosencephaly represents a complete lack of separation of the telencephalon. Presence of midline structures such as the falx excludes the diagnosis of alobar holoprosencephaly. The absence of the septum pellucidum is constant in holoprosencephaly, but may also be seen associated with other congenital abnormalities, including hydranencephaly. Severe hydrocephalus can closely mimic hydranencephaly, particularly on CT. The ventricles may be so enlarged that the brain is compressed into a thin mantle against the inside of the skull, and this mantle may be obscured by the beam hardening artifact that occurs with CT.

Teaching points

▶ Hydranencephaly is replacement of most of the supratentorial brain with large, thin-walled cystic spaces filled with CSF. The thalami and the cerebellum are preserved. The inferior medial frontal and temporal lobes and occipital lobes may be preserved as well.
▶ Hydranencephaly is thought to represent the result of a vascular (carotid occlusion) or infectious (toxoplasmosis or cytomegalovirus) insult occurring at a time of life when the response of the brain is to undergo liquefactive necrosis with minimal gliotic reaction.
▶ May be associated with microcephaly, normal head size, or even massive macrocephaly.

Next steps in management

MRI is helpful in distinguishing hydranencephaly from severe hydrocephalus, which has a much better prognosis after CSF shunting. Shunting may also be required for hydranencephaly to prevent massive macrocephaly, but is not necessary without increasing head size.

Further reading

1. Deeg KH, Gassner I. Sonographic diagnosis of brain malformations, part 2: holoprosencephaly—hydranencephaly—agenesis of septum pellucidum—schizencephaly—septo-optical dysplasia. Ultraschall Med. 2010 Dec;31(6):548–560.
2. Winter TC, Kennedy AM, Byrne J, Woodward PJ. The cavum septi pellucidi: why is it important? J Ultrasound Med. 2010 Mar;29(3):427–444.

History

▶ 4-year-old girl with right proptosis, erythema, and edema.

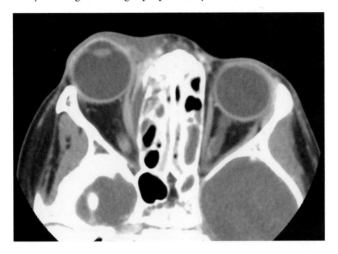

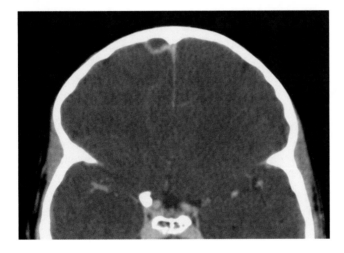

Case 95   Orbital Cellulitis Complicated by Subperiosteal and Epidural abscesses

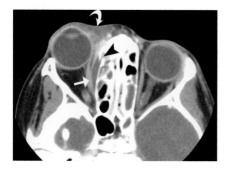 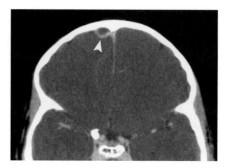

Findings

► Axial contrast-enhanced CT image (left) through the orbits shows right proptosis due to a subperiosteal abscess (arrow) adjacent to ethmoid sinusitis, causing lateral deviation of the medial rectus muscle. Note the defect in the lamina papyracea (arrowhead). Periorbital cellulitis (curved arrow) is also noted.

► Axial contrast-enhanced image (right) of the brain reveals a small epidural abscess (arrowhead).

Differential diagnosis

See below.

Teaching points

► Orbital infections are categorized based on their relationship to the orbital septum. The orbital septum is a thin band of fibrous tissue that extends between the orbital periosteum to the palpebral tissues that serves as a barrier to the spread of infection into the orbit.

► Preseptal, or periorbital, infections are due to spread of infection from the ocular adnexa, teeth, or the face and may be treated with oral antibiotics.

► Postseptal or orbital cellulitis results from the spread of sinusitis. The same complications can occur as are seen in other forms of sinusitis, such as mastoiditis, including thrombosis of the superior ophthalmic vein or cavernous sinus, and subperiosteal or epidural abscess, or meningitis. Postseptal infections require IV antibiotic therapy and the complications may require surgery.

Next steps in management

CT and MR are both suitable for the evaluation for complications. CT is more readily available on an urgent basis. Postseptal cellulitis requires IV antibiotic therapy. Subperiosteal abscess may require surgery. Epidural abscesses require neurosurgical consultation.

Further reading

1. Capps EF, Kinsella JF, Gupta M, et al. Emergency imaging assessment of acute, non-traumatic conditions of the head and neck. Radiographics. 2010;30:1335–1352.
2. LeBedis CA, Sakai O. Nontraumatic orbital conditions: diagnosis with CT and MR imaging in the emergent setting. Radiographics. 2008;28:1741–1753.

History

▶ 2-day-old term infant with low Apgar scores and metabolic acidosis.

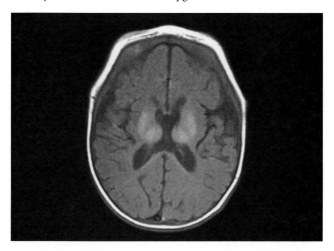

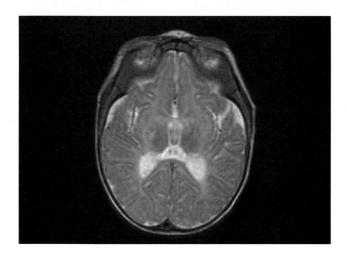

Case 96   Profound Hypoxic Ischemic Injury (HII)

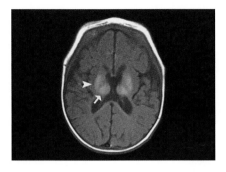 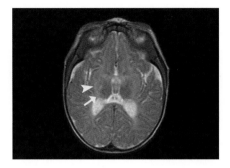

Findings

▶ Axial T1-weighted (left) and axial T2-weighted (right) images show abnormal hyperintense signal in the ventrolateral thalami (arrow) and posterolateral putamina (arrowhead).

Differential diagnosis

If the patient presents in the first 24 hours of life, HII is most likely, but if symptoms arise later in the perinatal period, the differential diagnostic considerations include meningitis, hypoglycemia, kernicterus, and metabolic disorders.

Teaching points

▶ Hypoxia and hypotension both cause brain injury in infants. The pattern of injury depends on the severity and duration of the insult as well as on the degree of brain maturation. The imaging appearance also depends upon the timing of imaging relative to the inciting event.

▶ In mild to moderate insults, blood is shunted to vital structures and the cortical and subcortical portions of the boundary or "watershed" zones between arterial territories are affected. For term infants, these are the parasagittal border zones as in older children and adults. For premature infants (<36 weeks), the boundary zone is the periventricular white matter and the resulting injury is periventricular leukomalacia.

▶ Profound insults primarily affect regions of high metabolic activity, which are also the areas of early myelination. In all infants, these include the posterolateral putamina, ventrolateral thalami, posterior limb of the internal capsule, perirolandic gyri, posterior brainstem, corona radiata, and cerebellar vermis.

▶ In profound perinatal hypoxia/hypotension MRI obtained within the first 24 hours may show normal findings on conventional images but reduced diffusion on diffusion-weighted sequences (DWI) and a lactate peak on MR spectroscopy (at 1.3 ppm at 1.5T) in affected areas. Early in the first week, T1- and T2-hyperintensity is observed in affected areas, but later in the first week or early second week, T2-shortening is noted.

Next steps in management

Follow-up MRI helps determine prognosis.

Further reading

1. Huang BY, Castillo M. Hypoxic-ischemic brain injury: Imaging findings from birth to adulthood. Radiographics. 2008 Mar–Apr;28(2):417–439.
2. Chao CP, Zaleski CG, Patton AC. Neonatal hypoxic-ischemic encephalopathy: multimodality imaging findings. Radiographics. 2006 Oct;26 Suppl 1:S159–S172.

History

▶ 2-year-old with developmental delay.

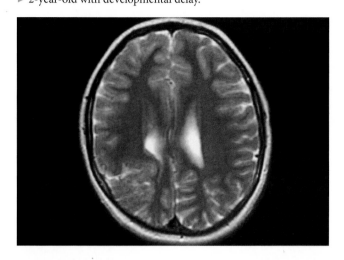

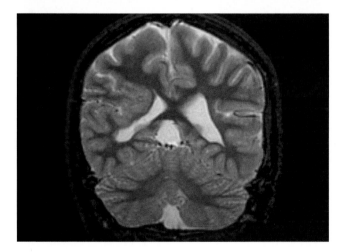

Case 97 Polymicrogyria

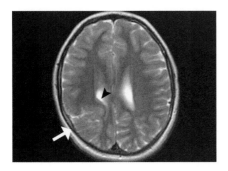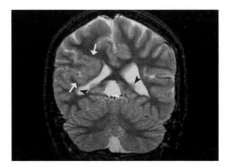

Findings

▶ Axial (left) and coronal (right) T2-weighted MR images show focal cortical thickening (arrows) posterior to the sylvian fissure with lack of normal underlying white matter and overlying sulci. The cortex is infolded or buckled toward the ventricle. Also noted are foci of nodular subependymal heterotopia (arrowheads).

Differential diagnosis

Thick cortex could also be due to pachygyria. Infolding or buckling of the cortex suggests closed-lip schizencephaly, but in polymicrogyria, the gray matter does not extend to the ependyma and the ventricle does not point to the abnormality.

Teaching points

▶ Polymicrogyria is a cortical malformation believed to occur in a late stage of cortical development. Polymicrogyria is considered a disorder of neuronal organization rather than of migration in which multiple tiny gyri are formed. Associated conditions include congenital infection (cytomegalovirus), in utero ischemia, or congenital syndromes (Aicardi syndrome).

▶ Polymicrogyria may be focal, multifocal, or diffuse. The most commonly involved site is the perisylvian region. The imaging appearance can be categorized into three main types:

  ▪ Coarse or bumpy
  ▪ Fused smooth outer cortex
  ▪ Fine or delicate

▶ MR with 3D spoiled gradient-echo acquisition is best for showing cortical abnormalities. Surface coils may be helpful in some cases. In general, there is lack of normal sulci and the cortex appears thick with irregular inner and outer surfaces. The cortex may follow the normal course or may buckle inward. The underlying white matter is gliotic and the imaging appearance depends on the degree of myelination of the surrounding white matter. Anomalous venous drainage is common and may provide a clue to an adjacent cortical malformation.

▶ Associated anomalies are common and include dysgenesis of the corpus callosum, cerebellar hypoplasia, and gray matter heterotopia.

Next steps in management

Associated additional anomalies and anomalous venous drainage should be sought on MR. Prognosis depends on the amount of cortex involved.

Further reading

1. Barkovich AJ. Current concepts of polymicrogyria. Neuroradiology. 2010 Jun;52(6):479–487.
2. Tarrant A, Garel C, Germanaud D, et al. Microcephaly: a radiological review. Pediatr Radiol. 2009 Aug;39(8):772–780.

Part 6　Chest and Airway

History

▶ Term fetus/infant with neck mass.

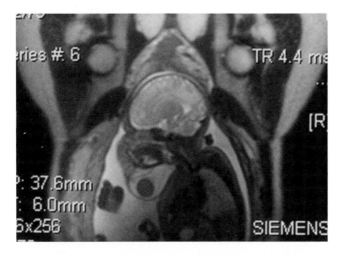

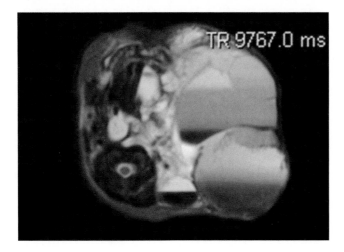

Case 98 Lymphatic Malformation (Lymphangioma) of Neck

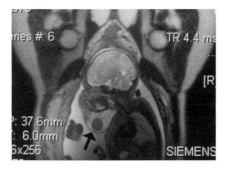 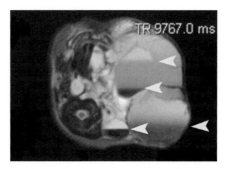

Findings

▶ Sagittal T2-weighted prenatal MR image (left) shows a mass with water and soft tissue intensity (arrow) involving the floor of the mouth and the neck.

▶ Axial postnatal T2-weighted MR image (right) shows a multilocular cystic mass with multiple fluid levels (arrowheads).

Differential diagnosis

The differential diagnosis for the cystic and solid mass on the prenatal exam also includes mature cystic teratoma. The finding of fat in the lesion would support the diagnosis of teratoma. If the structure were simply cystic, branchial cleft cyst could also be considered. The multilocular nature of the cystic mass and finding of fluid levels due to intralesional hemorrhage are characteristic of lymphatic malformation.

Teaching points

▶ Lymphatic malformation, also known as lymphangioma or cystic hygroma, is due to failure of development of channels that drain primordial lymph sacs. The cystic spaces can be distinguished as macro- or microcysts (macro larger than 1–2 cm) or as capillary, cavernous, or cystic.

▶ Lymphatic malformations can arise anywhere in the body, but common sites include the neck, floor of the mouth, axilla, and superior mediastinum. They typically dissect through fascial planes to involve many spaces. There is an association with Turner syndrome.

▶ Lymphatic malformations may be large enough to present at birth or they may present when they become symptomatic due to intralesional hemorrhage or infection. They also may undergo rapid periods of hormonally influenced growth at puberty and during pregnancy.

▶ Macrocystic components demonstrate fluid attenuation but may be complicated by infection or hemorrhage. Microcystic or capillary-sized cysts appear solid on imaging studies. Contrast enhancement is seen in the walls and septa of macrocystic components and in microcystic components.

Next steps in management

MRI and MRV are helpful in preoperative planning. Macrocystic components are best treated with ultrasound-guided sclerotherapy.

Further reading

1. Burrows PE, Laor T, Paltiel H, Robertson RL. Diagnostic imaging in the evaluation of vascular birthmarks. Dermatol Clin. 1998;16:455–488.
2. Koch BL. Cystic malformations of the neck in children. Pediatr Radiol.2005;35:463–477.

History

▶ 17-year-old with swelling near left mandibular angle.

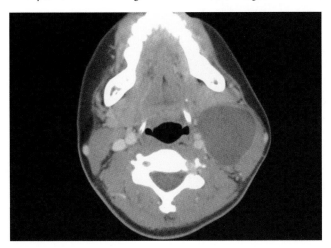

Case 99 Second Branchial Cleft Cyst

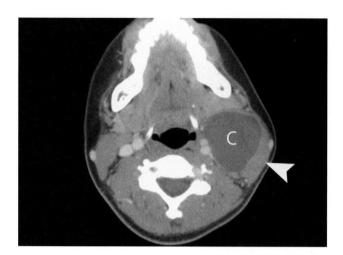

Findings

▶ Axial contrast-enhanced CT reveals a homogeneous, fluid-attenuation mass (C) just anterior and medial to the sternocleidomastoid muscle (arrowhead).

Differential diagnosis

The differential includes lateral cystic masses such as lymphatic malformation and suppurative or necrotic lymph nodes. Multiple septations would favor the former and adjacent confluent adenopathy would support the latter.

Teaching points

▶ Anomalous development of the branchial apparatus of the neck causes a spectrum of congenital abnormalities including cysts, fistulas, and sinuses. These may present at birth if large or later in childhood due to superinfection.
▶ First branchial cleft anomalies often occur near the external auditory canal and may involve the parotid gland.
▶ Second branchial cleft anomalies are most common. The most common location of the cyst is posterior to the submandibular gland, anteriomedial to the sternocleidomastoid muscle, and anterolateral to the carotid sheath.
▶ Third branchial cleft anomalies are rare and are most often fistulae to the pyriform sinus rather than cysts. Cysts are associated with the carotid sheath and a beak may extend between the carotid artery and jugular vein. Thymic cysts are a form of third cleft anomaly in which there is persistence of the thymopharyngeal duct, which is analogous to the thyroglossal duct.
▶ Fourth cleft anomalies are also rare and also connect to the pyriform sinus. The pyriform sinus fistula extends to the anterior lower neck near the thyroid gland. An abscess anterior to the left lobe of the thyroid gland suggests this anomaly.
▶ On imaging, the cyst may appear simple but infection may cause a complex appearance with increased attenuation of fluid, wall thickening, and surrounding inflammatory change. The cyst does not enhance unless infected, in which case rim-like enhancement is seen.

Next steps in management

Branchial cleft anomalies are treated surgically.

Further reading

1. Lev S, Lev MH. Imaging of cystic lesions. Radiol Clin North Am. 2000;38:113–127.
2. Koch BL. Cystic malformations of the neck in children. Pediatr Radiol. 2005;35:463–477.

History

▶ 3-month-old with stridor and choking with feeds.

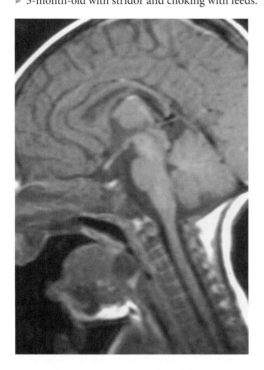

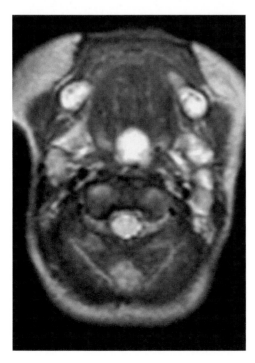

Case 100 Thyroglossal Duct Cyst at the Foramen Cecum

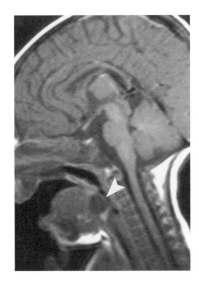 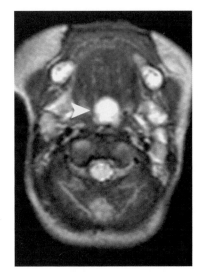

Findings

▶ Sagittal T1- (left) and axial T2-weighted (right) MR images (left) show a well-defined, fluid-intensity structure (arrowhead) with imperceptible wall at the midline base of the tongue.

Differential diagnosis

The differential diagnosis for the cystic midline lesions includes mature cystic teratoma and dermoid inclusion cyst. Both may contain fat and the former may contain calcifications. For base of tongue mass, the differential includes vallecular cyst and hemangioma.

Teaching points

▶ Thyroglossal duct cyst (TGDC) is the most common congenital mass of the neck. During fetal life, the thyroid anlage descends through the thyroglossal duct from the foramen cecum at the base of the tongue to the orthotopic position of the thyroid gland at the base of the neck. Aberrations of this process can result in cysts, fistulae, and ectopic thyroid tissue.

▶ Most TGDCs are asymptomatic and present due to superinfection.

▶ The majority of TGDCs are located in the midline, although they may be found in a paramedian location. Most (65%) are infrahyoid and usually located in the strap muscles. Ultrasound is the preferred imaging modality for midline neck mass in children. TGDCs often appear as simple cysts but may appear heterogeneously hypoechoic or even hyperechoic due to prior infection or hemorrhage. If infected at the time of diagnosis, the wall may appear thickened or indistinct. The cyst moves when the patient swallows.

▶ Thyroid carcinoma, usually papillary, develops in about 1% of TGDCs and is generally diagnosed in adults. The finding of calcification of a solid portion of the lesion is concerning for malignant transformation.

Next steps in management

Prior to surgery, the location of the thyroid gland should be determined with ultrasound and, if necessary, thyroid scintigraphy in order to prevent inadvertent total thyroidectomy. Treatment consists of resection of the cyst and the midportion of the hyoid bone.

Further reading

1. Lev S, Lev MH. Imaging of cystic lesions. Radiol Clin North Am. 2000;38:113–127.
2. Koch BL. Cystic malformations of the neck in children. Pediatr Radiol.2005;35:463–477.

History

► 4-year-old boy with 2-month history of sixth cranial nerve palsy.

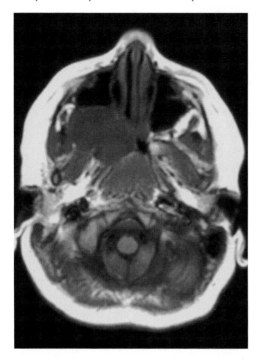

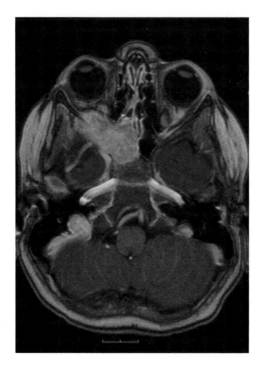

Case 101 Embryonal Rhabdomyosarcoma

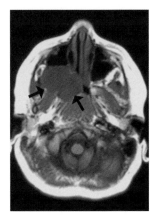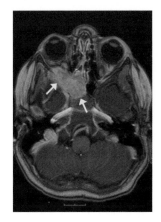

Findings

▶ Axial T1-weighted image (left) shows an expansile, intermediate-signal mass (arrows) centered on the pterygopalatine fossa and involving the posterior wall of the maxillary sinus.

▶ Post-gadolinium axial T1-weighted image (right) demonstrates diffuse enhancement of the mass (arrows), which involves the orbital apex causing bone destruction.

Differential diagnosis

The differential diagnosis of a solid mass about the head and neck includes vascular lesions such as infantile hemangioma in children less than 1 year of age and juvenile angiofibroma in adolescent boys. Rhabdomyosarcomas can be rather vascular as well. A distinguishing finding of rhabdomyosarcoma is bone erosion, which is seen in almost half of cases.

Teaching points

▶ Up to 40% of rhabdomyosarcomas occur in the head and neck. Sites of involvement are categorized into three types—the parameningeal sites (nasopharynx, pterygopalatine fossa, paranasal sinuses, middle ear, and orbit with bone erosion), non-parameningeal head and neck (parotid, oropharynx, cheek, neck), and the orbit without bone erosion. Parameningeal primary sites are associated with a worse prognosis.

▶ Embryonal rhabdomyosarcoma most frequently occurs in the first decade of life. The alveolar subtype is less common and occurs in adolescents.

▶ Rhabdomyosarcoma is an extremely aggressive tumor. Bone destruction, invasion of paranasal sinuses, perineural spread with intracranial extension, and spread to regional lymph nodes are common. CT demonstrates bone destruction quite well, while MR imaging is superior in demonstrating intracranial involvement. On CT, the mass is well defined, homogeneous, and isoattenuating to muscle. Necrosis and hemorrhage are common. Mild to moderate enhancement is noted.

▶ The mass is isointense to muscle on T1-weighted images and iso- to slightly hyperintense on T2-weighted images. Fat suppression is helpful for contrast-enhanced images for tumors of the face and orbit.

Next steps in management

Rhabdomyosarcoma is treated with multimodal therapy including surgical resection, radiation, and chemotherapy.

Further reading

1. Freiling NJ, Merks JH, Saeed P, et al. Imaging findings in craniofacial childhood rhabdomyosarcoma. Pediatr Radiol. 2010 Nov;40(11):1723–1738.
2. Robson CD. Imaging of head and neck neoplasms in children. Pediatr Radiol. 2010 Apr;40(4):499–509.

History

▸ 14-year-old with fever and sore throat.

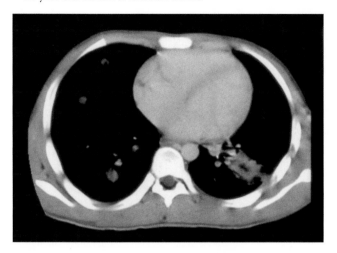

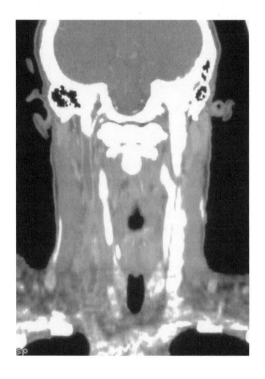

Case 102 Lemierre Syndrome—Septic Thrombosis of Jugular Vein with Septic Pulmonary Emboli

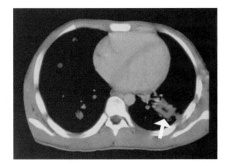 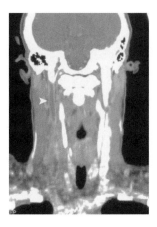

Findings

▶ CT of the chest (left) shows multiple pulmonary nodules and a wedge-shaped cavitary mass (arrow).

▶ Coronal CT angiogram (right) shows lack of luminal enhancement in the right internal jugular vein (arrowhead) with enhancement of the wall.

Differential diagnosis

The differential diagnosis of multiple pulmonary cystic or cavitary nodules in children includes metastatic disease, lymphoproliferative disorders, Langerhans cell histiocytosis, respiratory papillomatosis, infection (fungal infection, abscesses in patient with congenital immune deficiency), noninfectious inflammatory conditions (vasculitides), and tuberous sclerosis.

Teaching points

▶ Lemierre syndrome is an uncommon, serious condition resulting from septic thrombophlebitis of the jugular vein complicating an acute respiratory infection due to *Fusobacterium necroformans*. Patients, usually adolescents, present with symptoms of neck swelling and tenderness or of septic pulmonary emboli a week or two after symptoms of URI or tonsillitis. The eponym refers to thrombophlebitis of the jugular vein, but septic thrombophlebitis of adjacent veins may occur in any deep infection and should be sought on imaging studies.

▶ Imaging demonstrates no flow in a portion of the jugular vein. On CT with contrast, low attenuation of the lumen with enhancement of the wall is observed. On MR imaging, the signal intensity of the clot depends upon its age. Normally, a flow void is seen in the jugular vein.

▶ Septic pulmonary emboli are frequent. Findings on chest radiography typically include multiple, ill-defined, rounded or peripheral opacities, predominantly in the lower lungs. Nodules may be located at the end of a vessel and may be solid or cavitary.

Next steps in management

Lemierre syndrome is treated with aggressive antibiotic therapy. Anticoagulation may be used in cases of pulmonary emboli or involvement of dural venous sinuses.

Further reading

1. Capps EF, Kinsella JF, Gupta M, et al. Emergency imaging assessment of acute, non-traumatic conditions of the head and neck. Radiographics. 2010;30:1335–1352.
2. Weber AL, Siciliano A. CT and MR imaging evaluation of neck infections with clinical correlations. Radiol Clin North Am 2000;38(5):941–968, ix.

History

► 11-month-old with fever and dysphagia.

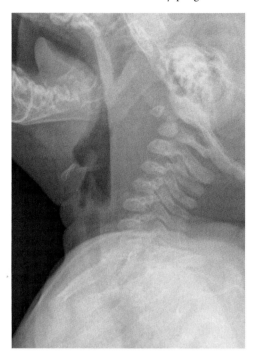

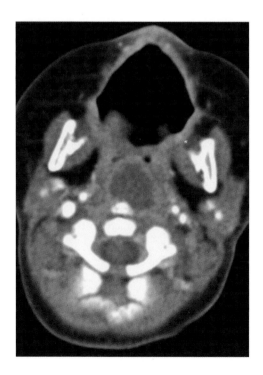

Case 103　Retropharyngeal Abscess

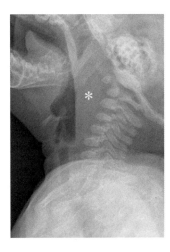 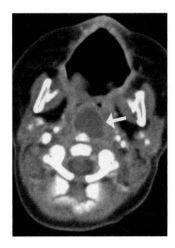

Findings

- ▶ Lateral soft-tissue neck radiograph (left) shows thickening of the retropharyngeal soft tissues (asterisk).
- ▶ Axial intravenous contrast-enhanced CT image (right) shows a well-defined, hypoattenuating mass (arrow) with rim-like, peripheral enhancement.

Differential diagnosis

The main differential consideration is retropharyngeal cellulitis, which is a deep infection requiring intravenous antibiotics, but which is treated medically, while retropharyngeal abscess usually requires surgical drainage. Cellulitis appears as soft-tissue thickening with hypoattenuation on CT due to edema, but without a fluid-attenuating mass with enhancing wall as seen with abscess.

Teaching points

- ▶ Retropharyngeal abscess most commonly occurs in children 6 to 12 months of age. In children the abscess results from the spread of bacterial pharyngitis or tonsillitis or rupture of suppurative adenitis.
- ▶ Children have short necks and redundant soft tissues, particularly with poor positioning and on expiratory radiographs. Lateral images are best obtained with a roll behind the shoulders to allow extension of the neck as young infants have relatively large heads. Airway fluoroscopy may help in cases of uncooperative patients.
- ▶ In young children, the normal soft tissues anterior to C2–3 may be as wide as the base of the vertebral body of C2. There is normally a step-off at C3, and the lower retropharyngeal soft tissues may be as wide as 1.5 vertebral bodies. Measurement is generally not necessary, as retropharyngeal swelling usually causes effacement of the normal step-off. Reversal of the normal cervical lordosis may also be noted.
- ▶ Complications should be sought on imaging and include extension to the superior mediastinum (be sure to scan down to the aortic arch), airway compression, jugular vein thrombosis, and carotid artery spasm or pseudo-aneurysm.

Next steps in management

Abscesses often require surgical drainage in addition to intravenous antibiotic therapy.

Further reading

1. Capps EF, Kinsella JF, Gupta M, et al. Emergency imaging assessment of acute, non-traumatic conditions of the head and neck. Radiographics. 2010;30:1335–1352.
2. Weber AL, Siciliano A. CT and MR imaging evaluation of neck infections with clinical correlations. Radiol Clin North Am 2000;38(5):941–968, ix.

History

▶ 6-month-old with enlarging facial mass.

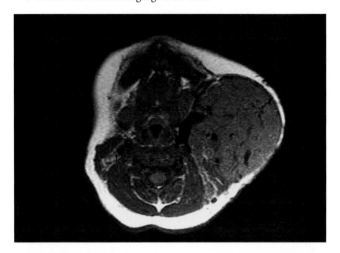

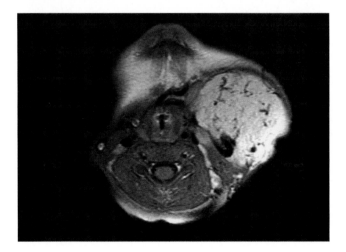

Case 104 Infantile Hemangioma

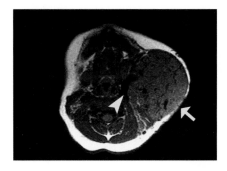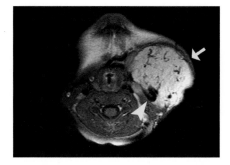

Findings

▸ Axial T1-weighted MR image (left) shows a large, lobulated, intermediate-signal mass (arrow) with large flow void (arrowhead).

▸ Post-gadolinium fat-suppressed T1-weighted MR image (right) shows homogeneous intense enhancement of the mass (arrow) with the exception of only the septa and vessels. Arrowhead indicates the flow void of the feeding artery.

Differential diagnosis

The differential diagnosis of a solid mass about the head and neck also includes rhabdomyosarcoma, which is not vascular, and malignant vascular tumors.

Teaching points

▸ Infantile hemangioma is a benign, high-flow vascular tumor. Hemangiomas are usually absent at birth and appear in the first few months of life. They have a characteristic natural history with a proliferative phase up to age 1 year followed by an involutional phase.

▸ If the hemangioma involves the skin, it has a characteristic appearance and is diagnosed clinically. Those that do not involve the skin come to imaging for diagnosis. Up to 50% of patients with hemangiomas have hemangiomas elsewhere, including the skin.

▸ Hemangiomas of the head and neck can occur anywhere but commonly involve the orbit, the face, and the parotid gland and rarely may occur in the subglottic trachea.

▸ The appearance on ultrasound is variable and nonspecific, but the vascular nature of the lesion is apparent with Doppler evaluation.

▸ Infantile hemangiomas may be diagnosed on the basis of their characteristic imaging appearance, obviating the need to biopsy a vascular tumor. On CT and MR, hemangiomas are very well marginated and separated into lobules by septations, which may contain vessels. They have very large feeding vessels at the periphery and enhance intensely and homogeneously except for the septations.

Next steps in management

Infantile hemangiomas do not require treatment unless they cause severe complications or if they involve the airway or the eye. Medical treatment may hasten involution.

Further reading

1. Burrows PE, Laor T, Paltiel H, Robertson RL. Diagnostic imaging in the evaluation of vascular birthmarks. Dermatol Clin 1998;16(3):455–488.
2. Paltiel HJ, Burrows PE, Kozakewich HP, et al. Soft-tissue vascular anomalies: utility of US for diagnosis. Radiology. 2000 Mar;214(3):747–754.

History

▶ 11-year-old with known diagnosis and shortness of breath.

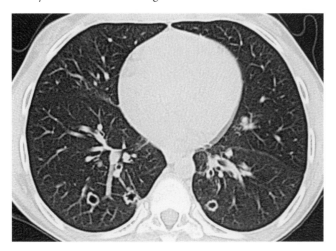

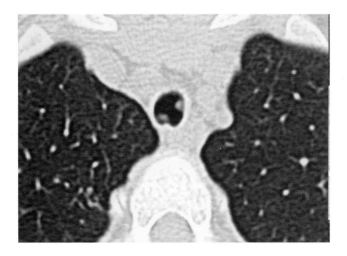

Case 105 Respiratory Papillomatosis Involving the Trachea and Lungs

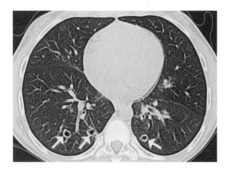 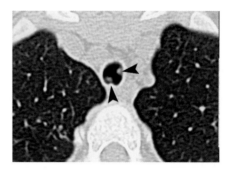

Findings

- ► Axial CT image of the chest (left) demsonstrates multiple bilateral cavitary nodules (arrows).
- ► Axial CT image (right) shows small polypoid projections along the wall of the trachea (arrowheads).

Differential diagnosis

The differential diagnosis of multiple cavitary nodules in children includes metastatic disease (rarely cavitary), lymphoproliferative disorders, Langerhans cell histiocytosis, infection (fungal infection, abscesses in an immunocompromised patient, septic pulmonary emboli), Wegener granulomatosis, and tuberous sclerosis.

Teaching points

- ► Laryngotracheal papillomatosis is caused by the human papilloma virus and the infection is acquired during passage through the birth canal. Most patients present with airway obstruction by age 4 years. Papillomas are the most common tracheal mass in children.
- ► Multiple surgical procedures are necessary to maintain a patent airway, and these rarely lead to dissemination of papillomas into the lungs through the bronchial tree. In the lungs, papillomas have a good blood supply and grow while destroying adjacent lung. The prognosis for children with pulmonary involvement is poor.
- ► If they survive childhood, there is a risk of malignant transformation to squamous cell carcinoma.
- ► Pulmonary involvement manifests as nodules of about 1 cm in diameter. These are solid and cavitary. Cavitary nodules may be thin- or thick-walled. Nodules are predominantly located in the posterior lower lobes.

Next steps in management

Disease is followed with plain radiographs and CT.

Further reading

1. Gélinas JF, Manoukian J, Côté A. Lung involvement in juvenile-onset recurrent respiratory papillomatosis: a systematic review of the literature. Int J Pediatr Otorhinolaryngol. 2008 Apr;72(4):433–452.
2. Kramer SS, Wehunt WD, Stocker JT, Kashima H. Pulmonary manifestations of juvenile laryngotracheal papillomatosis. AJR Am J Roentgenol. 1985 Apr;144(4):687–694.

History

▶ Newborn with respiratory distress and prenatal diagnosis.

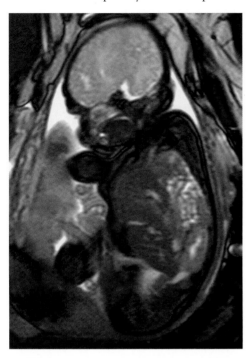

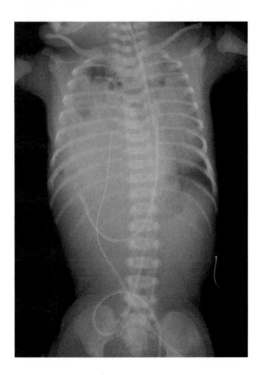

Case 106 Congenital Diaphragmatic Hernia (CDH)

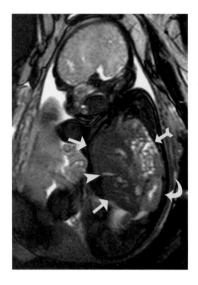 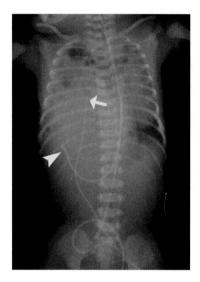

Findings

▶ Oblique sagittal T2-weighted prenatal MR image (left) shows the liver (arrows) extending through a gap in the diaphragm (arrowhead) into the thorax. Small bowel loops are seen posteriorly in the thorax (tailed arrow). The kidney (curved arrow) remains in the abdominal cavity.

▶ Postnatal AP radiograph (right) demonstrates soft-tissue-density and air-filled cystic structures representing bowel in the right thorax with shift of the mediastinal structures to the left. The orogastric tube tip (arrowhead) is deviated to the right and the umbilical venous catheter (arrow) courses above the diaphragm.

Differential diagnosis

Congenital lung malformations that may contain air should also be considered in the differential of an air-filled congenital chest mass. These include congenital pulmonary airway malformation and congenital lobar hyperinflation. These all start out opaque, then progressively fill with air as the baby breathes or swallows air.

Teaching points

▶ Failure of closure of the pleuroperitoneal canal allows bowel and other abdominal organs to enter the thorax, causing compression of the developing fetal lung. This compression inhibits branching and proliferation of airways and vessels, resulting in pulmonary hypoplasia. A large hernia causes shift of mediastinal structures and compromise of the contralateral lung as well.

▶ Up to 90% of CDHs are on the left and involve herniation of bowel. The stomach need not be herniated. On the right, the liver may herniate into the chest. Prognosis is much worse for these "liver-up" patients. Prenatal MRI is superior to ultrasound in quantifying the amount of herniated liver in fetuses with right-sided hernias, since liver and lung have similar echotexture.

Next steps in management

Initial management includes placement of a gastric tube to prevent distention of intrathoracic bowel loops.

Further reading

1. Schwartz DS, Reyes-Mugica M, Keller MS. Imaging of surgical diseases of the newborn chest. Radiol Clin North Am. 1999;37(6):1073–1077.
2. Jani JC, Cannie M, Peralta CF, et al. Lung volumes in fetuses with congenital diaphragmatic hernia: comparison of 3D US and MR imaging assessments. Radiology. 2007 Aug;244(2):575–582.

History

▶ 20-year-old female with shortness of breath.

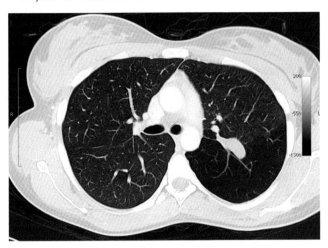

Case 107 Bronchial Atresia

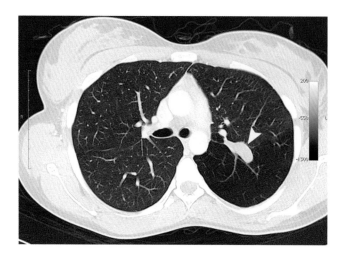

Findings

▸ CT image of the chest reveals a tubular, soft-tissue-attenuation structure (arrowhead) that is larger than adjacent vessels. The surrounding lung is hyperinflated.

Differential diagnosis

Solitary nodules in the lung in children are much more likely to be benign lesions or metastases than bronchogenic carcinoma. Benign lesions include congenital anomalies, arteriovenous malformation, and round pneumonia. Branching or tubular opacities suggest allergic bronchopulmonary aspergillosis or bronchial atresia. Adjacent hyperinflation indicates bronchial atresia.

Teaching points

▸ Bronchial atresia is caused by luminal occlusion of a bronchus thought to be due to an in utero vascular accident. Mucus accumulates in the lumen beyond the atresia, forming branched or tubular soft-tissue densities. These bronchi may or may not be dilated. The surrounding lung fills with some air from collateral drift, but the air is trapped by the bronchial atresia, so the lung served by the bronchus is slightly hyperinflated compared to normal lung.

▸ Bronchial atresia most commonly involves, in decreasing order of frequency, the left upper lobe, the right middle lobe, and the right upper lobe. These are the same sites of involvement of congenital lobar hyperinflation (CLH), but CLH is due to narrowing rather than occlusion of the bronchus. This allows air to get into the lung during inhalation when airways are wider due to negative pressure in the thorax. In exhalation, the airway becomes narrower, causing air to become trapped beyond the stenosis. As a result, in CLH the lobe overinflates, causing mass effect on the adjacent lobes and early presentation; in contrast, in bronchial atresia, only a small amount of air gets into the lobe via collateral drift, so there is only mild hyperinflation of the lobe and the condition is asymptomatic.

Next steps in management

Diagnosis is made on the basis of plain radiograph or CT.

Further reading

1. Hidekazu M, Noboru T, Masashi S, et al. Congenital bronchial atresia: radiologic findings in nine patients. J Comput Assist Tomogr. 2002;26:860–864
2. Newman B. Congenital bronchopulmonary foregut malformations: concepts and controversies. Pediatr Radiol. 2006;36: 773–791.

History

▶ 5-year-old with recurrent pneumonia.

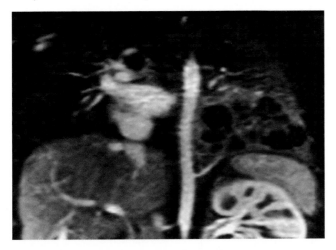

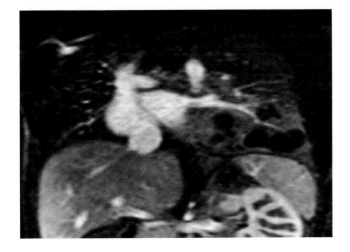

Case 108 Intralobar Pulmonary Sequestration

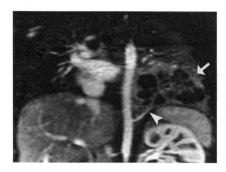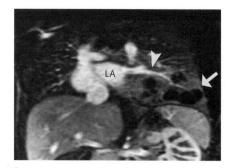

Findings

▶ Coronal MRA images demonstrate a mixed cystic and solid mass (arrow) in the left lower lobe with systemic arterial supply (arrowhead on left) and pulmonary venous drainage (arrowhead on right) to left atrium (LA).

Differential diagnosis

In a newborn, the differential diagnosis includes congenital pulmonary airway malformation (CPAM). In an older child the differential diagnosis includes infection.

Teaching points

▶ Pulmonary sequestration is defined as lung tissue with systemic arterial supply and no normal connection to the tracheal bronchial tree. Two types are defined:
  ▪ Extralobar—has its own pleural investment and occurs in or near the diaphragm (may be infra-diaphragmatic). Usually has systemic venous drainage. Ninety percent are on the left. Associated with other anomalies.
  ▪ Intralobar—shares pleura with adjacent lung. Usually pulmonary venous drainage. Almost always occurs in the lower lobe. May contain air.
▶ Extralobar sequestration commonly occurs as part of a hybrid lesion with small cyst CPAM. The features of different congenital malformations frequently overlap and they may all be considered part of a spectrum of bronchopulmonary–foregut malformations. Naming the lesion is less important than identifying important features for the surgeon, including systemic arterial supply, connection to the foregut, and associated anomalies.
▶ Extralobar sequestration is a congenital anomaly often identified prenatally. Intralobar sequestration commonly presents as recurrent lower lobe consolidation and may represent an acquired lesion due to chronic infection. Lack of oxygen exchange in the infected lung leads to shunting away of pulmonary flow and hypertrophy of systemic arterial supply. On the other hand, intralobar sequestrations are increasingly discovered in utero. It is possible that those discovered in older patients are congenital lesions that became infected.
▶ On prenatal ultrasound, sequestrations appear echogenic.

Next steps in management

Diagnosis is based on demonstration of systemic arterial supply. Treatment is surgical.

Further reading

1. Biyyam DR, Chapman T, Ferguson MR, et al. Congenital lung abnormalities: embryologic features, prenatal diagnosis, and post-natal radiologic pathologic correlation. Radiographics. 2010 Oct;30(6):1721–1738.
2. Newman B. Congenital bronchopulmonary foregut malformations: concepts and controversies. Pediatr Radiol. 2006;36: 773–791.

History

▶ 2-week-old with respiratory distress.

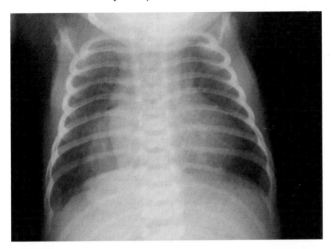

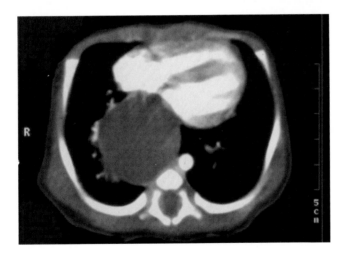

Case 109 Bronchogenic Cyst

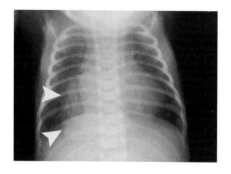 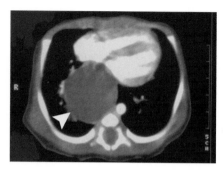

Findings

▶ PA chest radiograph demonstrates a large, round opacity posterior to the right heart (arrowheads).
▶ Contrast-enhanced CT image shows the mass (arrowhead) is of uniform fluid attenuation with an imperceptible wall and no enhancement or solid components.

Differential diagnosis

Other congenital lung malformations should also be considered, especially sequestration and congenital pulmonary airway malformation (CPAM). Sequestration is distinguished by systemic arterial supply and CPAM consists of more than one cyst, and these contain some air. Medial lung masses and posterior mediastinal masses are difficult to distinguish. An important differential consideration is neuroblastoma, which can be congenital. The finding of enhancing, soft-tissue components would favor neuroblastoma.

Teaching points

▶ Bronchogenic cysts are a type of bronchopulmonary foregut malformation. Approximately two thirds are located in the mediastinum and about one third are located in the medial lungs. The most common site is the subcarinal region.
▶ Large cysts may present in infancy, usually with respiratory distress. Smaller lesions are usually found incidentally on chest radiographs.
▶ Bronchogenic cysts do not communicate with the airway or contain air unless complicated by infection, in which case an air-fluid level may be noted. If the cyst compresses a bronchus, hyperinflation of the adjacent lung may be seen.
▶ On CT evaluation, bronchogenic cysts are homogeneous. The attenuation coefficient of the fluid may be up to 40 Hounsfield units due to the proteinaceous content of the fluid. The wall is imperceptible and the cyst does not enhance with intravenous contrast administration.
▶ On MR imaging, the cysts are hyperintense on T2-weighted images but of variable signal on T1-weighted images, depending on the protein content of the cyst fluid.

Next steps in management

Surgical resection is indicated for definitive diagnosis and to prevent complications, including hemorrhage and malignant transformation.

Further reading

1. Berrocal T, Madrid C, Novo S, et al. Congenital anomalies of the tracheobronchial tree, lung and mediastinum: embryology, radiology, and pathology. Radiographics 2003;24:e17–e62.
2. Patterson A. Imaging evaluation of congenital lung abnormalities in infants and children. Radiol Clin North Am. 2005; 43:303–323.

History

► 2-day-old with prenatal finding.

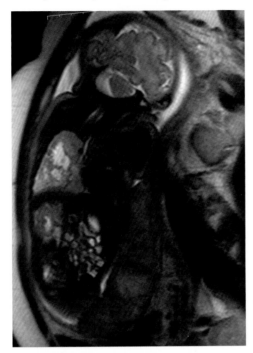

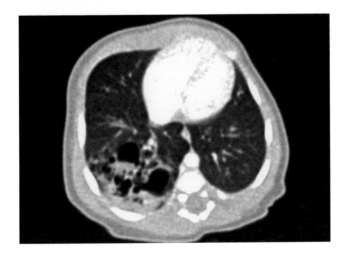

Case 110 Congenital Pulmonary Airway Malformation (CPAM)

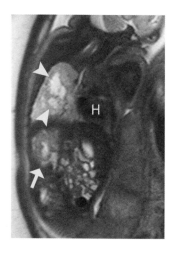
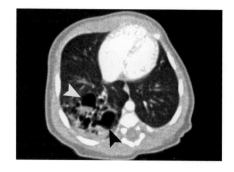

Findings

▶ Prenatal oblique coronal T2-weighted image (left) shows small cysts (arrowheads) in the right lung. Arrow indicates right kidney. (H = heart)

▶ Postnatal contrast-enhanced CT shows cystic-solid lesion in the right lung with air-containing cysts (arrowheads).

Differential diagnosis

In the newborn, consider other congenital thoracic abnormalities. After the neonatal period, the differential includes necrotizing pneumonia with abscess or pneumatoceles.

Teaching points

▶ CPAM was previously known as congenital cystic adenomatoid malformation.

▶ Stocker's original description of three histologic types has been expanded to five, although there are only three distinct radiographic appearances. Stocker type IV overlaps with the predominantly cystic form of pleuropulmonary blastoma (type 1 PPB). Type I, the most common type, consists of a large cyst surrounded by smaller cysts. Type II is formed of multiple smaller cysts. Type III is composed of microcysts and appears solid on imaging. To limit confusion in nomenclature, some authors advocate describing the three distinct radiologic appearances as large cyst (Stocker type I or IV), small cyst (type II), and microcystic (type III). Large cyst CPAM is indistinguishable from type I PPB.

▶ At birth CPAMs are filled with fluid and may appear solid. Due to an abnormal connection to the airway, the fluid is slow to clear, but is replaced by air. The fluid- and air-filled cysts have similar attenuation to normal lung that contains air and vessels, so lesions may be missed on supine radiographs.

Next steps in management

If discovered prenatally, CT is indicated. Systemic arterial supply should be sought in small cyst lesions. Iodinated contrast facilitates low-dose technique. Symptomatic patients undergo resection. Those lesions that are found prenatally but decrease in size are followed and resected if they fail to resolve.

Further reading

1. Biyyam DR, Chapman T, Ferguson MR, et al. Congenital lung abnormalities: embryologic features, prenatal diagnosis, and post-natal radiologic pathologic correlation. Radiographics. 2010 Oct;30(6):1721–1738.
2. Schwartz DS, Reyes-Mugica M, Keller MS. Imaging of surgical diseases of the newborn chest. Radiol Clin North Am. 1999 Nov;37(6):1067–1078.

History

▶ Newborn with respiratory distress. Second image obtained 2 days later.

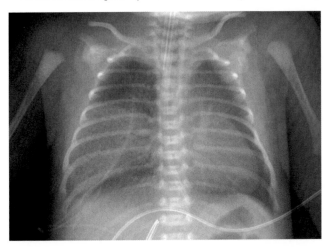

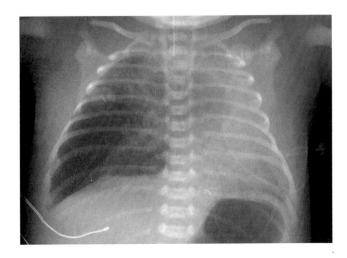

Case 111 Congenital Lobar Hyperinflation (CLH)

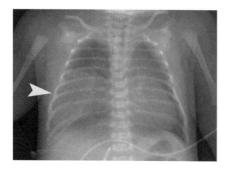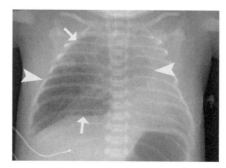

Findings

▶ AP chest radiograph of the newborn (left) shows an endotracheal tube and hyperexpanded but dense right middle lobe (arrowhead).

▶ Chest radiograph obtained 2 days later (right) shows increased expansion of the right middle lobe (arrowheads), which is now hyperlucent and extends across the midline. Atelectasis of the left lung and right upper and lower lobes (arrows) is now observed.

Differential diagnosis

CLH may be mistaken for pneumothorax, but the configuration of an expanded lobe, lack of collapsed lung at the hilum, and lung markings distinguish CLH. Another consideration in the neonate is large cyst congenital pulmonary airway malformation.

Teaching points

▶ Congenital lobar hyperinflation, except for the rare polyalveolar variant, is not a specific malformation, but the result of bronchial narrowing. This narrowing may be due to an intrinsic abnormality such as bronchostenosis or may be due to extrinsic compression, for example by a crossing vessel. The latter likely explains the association with congenital heart disease.

▶ The abnormality usually affects one of the upper lobes or the right middle lobe.

▶ Airways are slightly larger in inhalation, due to the negative pressure in the chest. Due to the narrowing of the bronchus in CLH, air is able to enter the lobe in inhalation but not to leave in exhalation, leading to progressive over-expansion of the lobe. The narrowed bronchus also causes delay in the clearance of lung fluid postnatally, so the lobe is initially opaque but becomes progressively more lucent.

▶ On CT, the over-expanded, radiolucent lobe is seen to contain attenuated vessels at the periphery of alveoli and no soft-tissue components. CT is helpful to evaluate for an extrinsic cause such as mediastinal mass.

Next steps in management

Symptomatic patients require surgical resection.

Further reading

1. Biyyam DR, Chapman T, Ferguson MR, et al. Congenital lung abnormalities: embryologic features, prenatal diagnosis, and post-natal radiologic pathologic correlation. Radiographics. 2010 Oct;30(6):1721–1738.
2. Patterson A. Imaging evaluation of congenital lung abnormalities in infants and children. Radiol Clin North Am. 2005; 43:303–323.

History

▶ Newborn with tachypnea after G-tube placement. Lateral view at age 8 months.

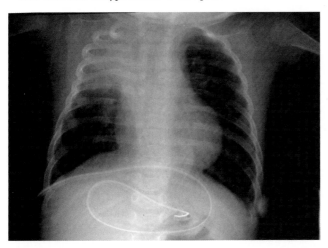

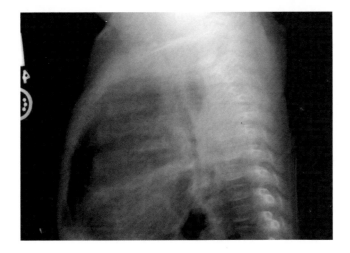

Case 112 Tracheal Bronchus/Tracheomalacia Associated with Esophageal Atresia

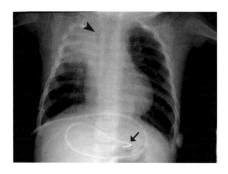 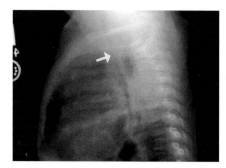

Findings

▶ PA chest radiograph (left) demonstrates atelectasis of the right upper lobe and an air bronchogram of a tracheal bronchus (arrowhead). Also noted is a G-tube (arrow), which was placed prior to delayed repair of esophageal atresia.

▶ Lateral radiograph (right) obtained after the esophageal atresia repair shows narrowing of the trachea (arrow).

Differential diagnosis

Tracheal stenosis.

Teaching points

▶ Tracheal bronchus (bronchus suis) is a bronchus serving usually the right upper lobe that originates directly from the trachea. Tracheal bronchus is associated with esophageal atresia. Patients may present with recurrent upper lobe pneumonia or air trapping or with upper lobe atelectasis after endotracheal intubation beyond the origin of the tracheal bronchus.

▶ Tracheomalacia is collapse of the trachea in exhalation due to soft cartilage rings. All infants have some degree of tracheal softening, which resolves with advancing age, but significant tracheal obstruction is abnormal. This condition is associated with esophageal atresia and vascular rings. Dynamic imaging with fluoroscopy confirms the diagnosis. Tracheomalacia resolves by age 2 to 3 years.

▶ Tracheal stenosis is a fixed narrowing of the trachea that may be long or short segment, congenital or acquired usually secondary to prolonged intubation. In congenital tracheal stenosis, the narrowing of the lumen is due to the presence of complete or O-shaped rather than C-shaped cartilage rings, is associated with pulmonary sling, and imparts a poorer prognosis.

Next steps in management

Treatment for tracheomalacia is to treat symptoms until resolution. Esophagram is indicated for stenosis to evaluate for pulmonary sling. Tracheal bronchus may require surgery if complicated by recurrent infection. MDCT is helpful for preoperative planning.

Further reading

1. Berrocal T, Madrid C, Novo S, et al. Congenital anomalies of the tracheobronchial tree, lung, and mediastinum: embryology, radiology, and pathology. Radiographics. 2004 January;24:e17.
2. Lee EY, Boiselle PM, Shamberger RC. MDCT and 3-dimensional imaging: preoperative evaluation of thoracic vascular and tracheobronhcial anomalies in pediatric patients. J Pediatr Surg. 2010 Apr;45(4):811–821.

History

▶ 16-month-old with fever, tachypnea, and cough, worsening despite oral antibiotic therapy.

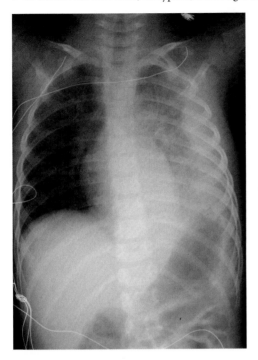

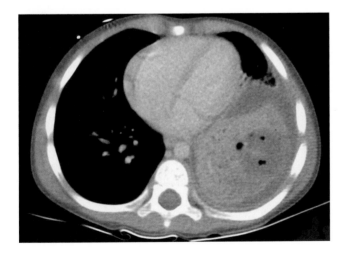

Case 113 Pneumonia Complicated by Empyema and Abscess

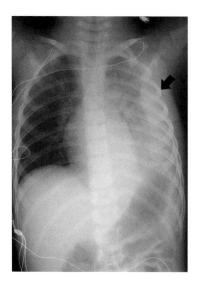 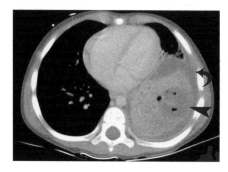

Findings

▶ Upright frontal radiograph shows near-complete opacification of the left hemithorax with lateral pleural-based density tracking along the chest wall (arrow).

▶ CT shows consolidated lung with a fluid- and air-filled cavity within (arrowhead) and adjacent nondependent pleural fluid collection (curved arrow).

Differential diagnosis

Other causes of near-complete opacification of a hemithorax are less common and include the following:

▶ Pulmonary contusion and large hemothorax
▶ Ewing sarcoma of rib
▶ Pleuropulmonary blastoma

Teaching points

▶ After the neonatal period, pneumonia in children, like adults, is usually lobar. Near-complete opacification of the hemithorax suggests complicated pneumonia with empyema.

▶ The most common causative pathogens are pneumococcus and *Staphylococcus aureus*.

▶ Air-filled cavities may be seen on imaging and may represent abscess, cavitary necrosis, or pneumatocele.

▶ On contrast-enhanced CT, consolidated lung enhances while necrotic lung does not, but in both cases, the prognosis is good following drainage of the adjacent empyema and treatment with intravenous antibiotics.

Next steps in management

Treatment with intravenous antibiotics alone is insufficient. Drainage of the empyema by a surgeon or interventional radiologist with mechanical or fibrinolytic disruption of the multiple septations within the fluid collection is required. CT or ultrasound may be used for guidance.

Further reading

1. Donnelly LF. Imaging in immunocompetent children who have pneumonia. Radiol Clin North Am. 2005 Mar;43(2):253–265.
2. Lewis RA, Feigin RD. Current issues in the diagnosis and management of pediatric empyema. Semin Pediatr Infect Dis. 2002 Oct;13(4):280–288.

History

▶ 18-month-old with acute shortness of breath 3 days ago, now clinically improved.

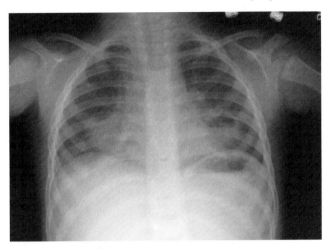

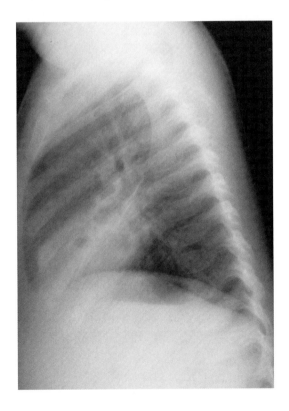

Case 114 Pneumatoceles in Hydrocarbon Pneumonitis

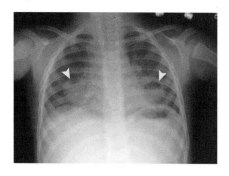 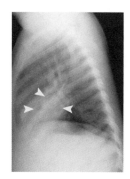

Findings

▶ PA and lateral chest radiographs demonstrate fluffy bilateral opacities in the right middle lobe and lingula containing air-filled cavities (arrowheads).

Differential diagnosis

The differential diagnosis for air-filled cavities also includes pulmonary abscess and cavitary pulmonary necrosis. Clinical status helps to differentiate necrosis and abscess, in which the patient is sick, from pneumatocele, in which the patient is clinically improving. Other clues indicating severe infection, such as near white-out of the lung and large nondependent pleural fluid collection, would suggest necrotizing pneumonia or abscess. On CT, abscesses tend to have thick, irregular walls, while pneumatoceles have smooth, thin walls. Abscesses would be found in enhancing consolidated lung, while cavitary necrosis is seen in lung tissue that is nonenhancing. Differentiating the abscess from cavitary necrosis is not clinically important as both do well in the long term with drainage of the empyema and intravenous antibiotic therapy.

Teaching points

▶ Pneumatoceles in children may be caused by a number of disparate conditions, including the following:
  ▪ Hydrocarbon aspiration
  ▪ Pneumonia—*S. aureus*, pneumococcus, tuberculosis
  ▪ Langerhans cell histiocytosis
  ▪ Pulmonary contusion
▶ Pneumatoceles are thought to result from alveolar rupture into an inflamed interstitium. They generally resolve in 1 to 2 months and have no prognostic significance.
▶ Household hydrocarbons include furniture and floor polish, gasoline, kerosene, and lighter fluid. They have a very low viscosity and are therefore easily aspirated if swallowed. Vomiting should not be induced as vomiting hydrocarbons increases the chance of aspiration. Hydrocarbons cause an intense chemical pneumonitis and destroy surfactant, causing diffuse alveolar collapse. Radiographs will demonstrate abnormalities within 12 hours of the aspiration. Diffuse patchy consolidations appear in the lower and right middle lobes.

Next steps in management

Hydrocarbon aspiration is self-limited and treated supportively.

Further reading

1. Donnelly LF. Imaging in immunocompetent children who have pneumonia. Radiol Clin North Am. 2005;43:253–265.
2. Seely JM, Effmann EL. Acute lung injury and acute respiratory distress syndrome in children. Semin Roentgenol. 1998 Apr;33(2):163–173.

History

▶ 5-year-old with fever and cough.

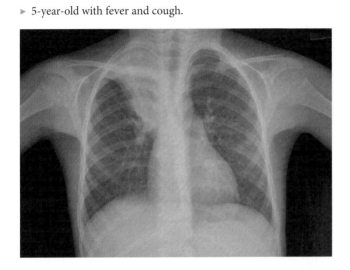

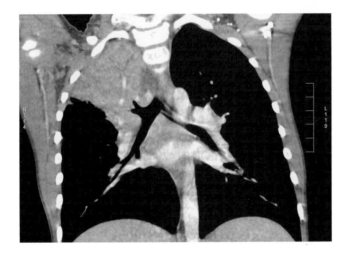

Case 115   Mycoplasma Pneumonia Mimicking Primary Tuberculosis

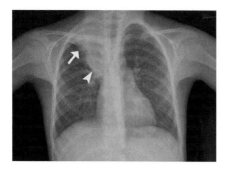 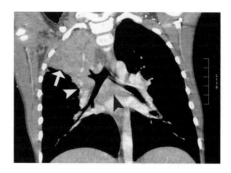

Findings

▸ PA radiograph (left) shows opacification and partial collapse of the right upper lobe (arrow) with a rounded configuration at the lower margin of the collapse due to unilateral hilar adenopathy (arrowhead). This is the "Golden S" sign.

▸ Coronal reformation of a contrast-enhanced CT scan shows consolidated partially collapsed upper lobe (arrow) and hilar (white arrowhead) and subcarinal (black arrowhead) adenopathy.

Differential diagnosis

Unilateral hilar adenopathy should be considered to represent primary tuberculosis until proved otherwise. Adenopathy can lead to lobar collapse. Adenopathy and lobar consolidation due to *Mycobacterium tuberculosis* is called the "primary" or "Ranke" complex. Parahilar and subcarinal adenopathy may also be noted. Small pleural effusion is common with primary tuberculosis. On CT, lymph nodes may be hypoattenuating due to central caseating necrosis. Patients are often immunocompromised (e.g., HIV disease).

   Chronic inhaled foreign body should also be considered with the findings of atelectasis and hilar adenopathy. Bronchoscopy may be necessary to arrive at a final diagnosis.

Teaching points

▸ *Mycoplasma pneumoniae* is the most common cause of pulmonary infection in children. School-age children are most often affected.

▸ Early radiographic findings include fine reticular opacities, which are usually unilateral and segmental in distribution. With more advanced disease, fluffy confluent opacities similar to those seen in bacterial infection are observed. Hilar adenopathy is common. Small pleural effusion may be noted.

▸ High-resolution CT may also demonstrate a tree-in-bud appearance similar to that seen in cystic fibrosis.

▸ Mycoplasma pneumonia may be complicated by obliterative bronchiolitis.

Next steps in management

The patient should be put into respiratory isolation immediately until tuberculosis is excluded with skin testing and evaluation of sputum or bronchial washings for acid-fast bacilli.

Further reading

1. Fonseca-Santos J. Tuberculosis in children. Eur J Radiol. 2005 Aug;55(2):202–208.
2. Herold CJ, Sailer JG. Community-acquired and nosocomial pneumonia. Eur Radiol. 2004 Mar;14 Suppl 3:E2–E20.

History

▶ 16-year-old with fever and worsening cough.

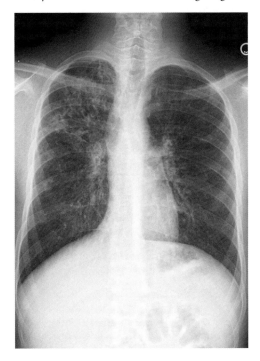

Case 116   Cystic Fibrosis

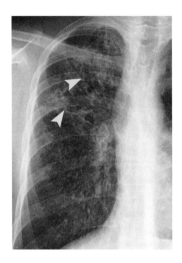

Findings

► PA chest radiograph (previous page) demonstrates upper lobe-predominant increased interstitial markings with upper lobe bronchiectasis (arrowheads). Right paratracheal adenopathy is also noted.

Differential diagnosis

The differential diagnosis of bronchiectasis includes recurrent aspiration, chronic foreign body aspiration, allergic bronchopulmonary aspergillosis, primary ciliary dyskinesia, and congenital or acquired immunodeficiency syndromes.

Teaching points

► Cystic fibrosis (CF) is the most common lethal genetic disease of white children. CF is a multisystem disease characterized by abnormally viscous secretions.
► Most present in early childhood with chronic recurrent respiratory infections or wheezing. Others present with GI symptoms including constipation, malabsorption, and failure to thrive. Up to 20% present in the neonatal period with meconium ileus (see Case 27).
► Early chest radiographic findings consist of air-trapping and mild bronchial wall thickening mimicking viral infection or reactive airways disease.
► Later findings include marked bronchial wall thickening and bronchiectasis, initially with upper lobe predominance. Other findings include small nodular opacities and mucoid impaction.
► Late findings include enlarged hila due to lymphadenopathy and/or pulmonary arterial enlargement from pulmonary hypertension. Cor pulmonale occurs in the end-stage. Older patients may develop life-threatening hemoptysis from enlarged systemic arteries.
► HRCT is valuable in the detection of early focal disease in patients with normal pulmonary function tests and also in monitoring response to therapy.

Next steps in management

Diagnosis is based on a positive sweat chloride test. Comparison to prior exams helps in diagnosis of acute infections.

Further reading

1. Moskowitz SM, Gibson RL, Effmann EL. Cystic fibrosis lung disease: genetic influences, microbial interactions, and radiological assessment. Pediatr Radiol. 2005 Aug;35(8):739–757.
2. Javidan-Nejad C, Bhalla S. Bronchiectasis. Radiol Clin North Am. 2009 Mar;47(2):289–306.

History

▶ 9-year-old boy with chest pain and shortness of breath.

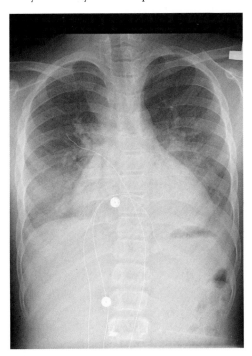

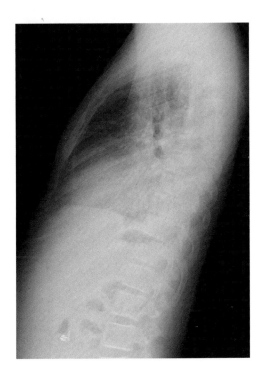

Case 117 Sickle Cell Anemia with Acute Chest Syndrome

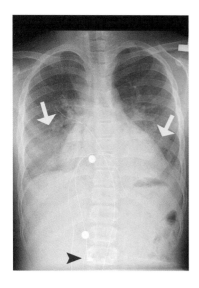 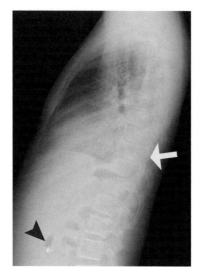

Findings

▶ PA and lateral chest radiographs demonstrate an enlarged cardiac silhouette, bibasilar consolidations (arrows) with obscuration of the left hemidiaphragm and the posterior right hemidiaphragm with likely small effusions. Also noted are cholecystectomy clips (arrowheads). No spleen shadow is seen.

Differential diagnosis

Bilateral consolidations with small effusions could also represent pneumonia in a normal child, but the additional findings of cardiomegaly, history of cholecystectomy, and lack of a spleen impression on the stomach indicate the underlying condition of sickle cell anemia.

Teaching points

▶ Acute chest syndrome (ACS) is the development of a new consolidation in a patient with sickle cell anemia presenting with fever, chest pain, dyspnea, and/or wheezing.

▶ Consolidations may be solitary or multiple and bilateral, usually involve the lower lung zones, and are frequently associated with small pleural effusions. The radiographic findings may progress rapidly and follow-up radiographs are helpful if initial images are unrevealing in a patient with clinical suspicion of ACS.

▶ Other radiographic findings of sickle cell anemia help to narrow the differential if this history is not provided. Such findings include:

▪ Cardiomegaly from chronic anemia
▪ Absence of spleen shadow
▪ Cholecystectomy for pigment gallstone disease
▪ Avascular necrosis of humeral heads
▪ H-shaped vertebral bodies due to infarction of the ossification centers of the end plates

Next steps in management

As respiratory infection is commonly associated with ACS, antibiotic therapy is used. Additional modalities, including plasma exchange and nitric oxide therapy, may be required.

Further reading

1. Vij R, Machado RF. Pulmonary complications of hemoglobinopathies. Chest. 2010 Oct;138(4):973–983.
2. Quinn CT, Buchanan GR. The acute chest syndrome of sickle cell disease. J Pediatr. 1999 Oct;135(4):416–422.

History

► 19-month-old girl with fever and cough.

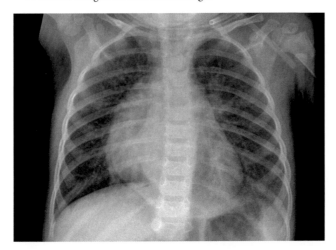

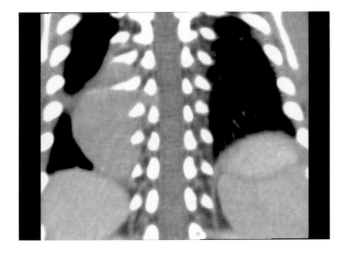

Case 118 Posterior Mediastinal Neuroblastoma

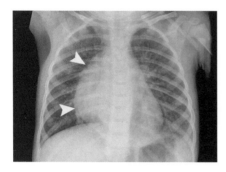 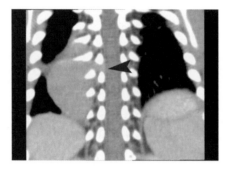

Findings

▶ PA chest radiograph (left) shows right lower lobe consolidation and paraspinal mass (arrowheads).
▶ Coronal CT reformat shows elongate paraspinal tumor with subtle neural foraminal invasion (arrowhead).

Differential diagnosis

Differential includes other ganglion cell tumors, but the age makes neuroblastoma the most likely diagnosis.

Teaching points

▶ The thorax is the second most common site of origin for neuroblastoma after the abdomen.
▶ Mean age at presentation for neuroblastoma is 22 months. Ganglioneuroblastoma and ganglioneuroma generally occur in older patients. Clinical presentation is highly variable.
  ▪ Blueberry muffin syndrome—violaceous skin nodules
  ▪ Pepper syndrome—respiratory distress due to an enlarged liver with metastases
  ▪ Hutchinson syndrome—bone pain due to metastatic disease
  ▪ Raccoon eyes—discoloration of the periorbital regions due to orbital metastases; mimics child abuse
  ▪ Opsoclonus-myoclonus (dancing eyes, dancing feet/cerebellar ataxia)—probably a paraneoplastic syndrome
  ▪ Diarrhea due to tumoral secretion of vasoactive intestinal peptide (VIP)
  ▪ Horner syndrome—superior sulcus tumor
▶ Tumors at the thoracolumbar junction are particularly prone to extend through the neural foramina to invade the spinal canal. In the posterior mediastinum and retroperitoneum, neuroblastic or ganglion cell tumors tend to grow along the sympathetic chain in a craniocaudal direction and have an elongate appearance seen best on coronal and sagittal images.
▶ Neuroblastoma in the posterior mediastinum may cause splaying or erosion of adjacent ribs or erosion of pedicles or posterior scalloping of the vertebral bodies if the tumor extends into the spinal canal.

Next steps in management

MR or CT shows local extent of tumor. MR better shows spinal canal involvement. Catecholamine analog scintigraphy with metaiodobenzyl-guanidine (MIBG) or somatostatin analog is useful in evaluation for distant metastases. Bone scintigraphy shows bone metastases.

Further reading

1. Lonergan GJ, Schwab CM, Suarez ES, Carlson CL. Neuroblastoma, ganglioneuroblastoma, and ganglioneuroma: radiologic-pathologic correlation. Radiographics. 2002 Jul–Aug;22(4):911–934.
2. Restrepo CS, Eraso A, Ocazionez D, et al. The diaphragmatic crura and retrocrural space: normal imaging appearance, variants, and pathologic conditions. Radiographics. 2008 Sep–Oct;28(5):1289–1305.

History

▶ 3-year-old girl with fever, cough, and shortness of breath.

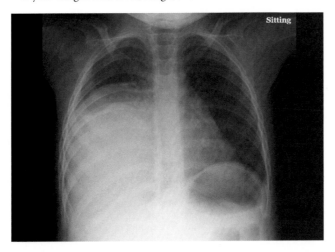

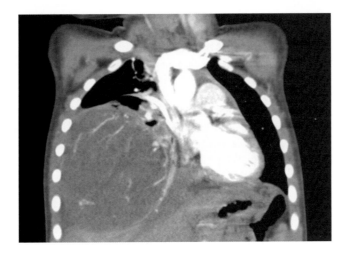

Case 119 Pleuropulmonary Blastoma (PPB)

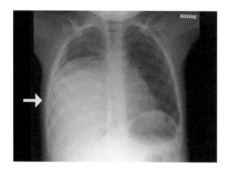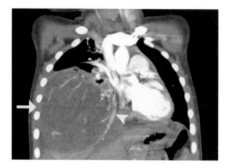

Findings

▶ PA chest radiograph (left) shows a large mass (arrow) in the right lower thorax that silhouettes the right hemidiaphragm and right heart border.

▶ Coronal contrast-enhanced CT reformat demonstrates that the mass (arrow) is hypoattenuating to muscle and contains some nontapering, enhancing vessels. Arrowhead = compressed lung.

Differential diagnosis

A large thoracic mass could also represent a chest wall mass such as Ewing sarcoma or Askin tumor (chest wall primitive neuroectodermal tumor) or a posterior mediastinal ganglion cell series mass, such as neuroblastoma or ganglioneuroblastoma. Inflammatory myofibroblastic tumors most commonly arise in the lung and may be large, but generally not this large. Large, chunky calcifications are common.

Teaching points

▶ Although rare, PPB is the most common primary lung tumor in children. Bronchogenic carcinoma is exceedingly rare in children and is only encountered in older children. Pediatric PPB is a small round blue cell tumor that is histologically indistinguishable from Wilms' tumor. Pediatric PPB is not the same disease as the tumor with the same name that occurs in adults, in that only the sarcomatous and blastematous elements are malignant in the pediatric form. The epithelial components are benign.

▶ There are three types:

  ▪ Type I—Purely cystic—radiologically indistinguishable from type 1 congenital pulmonary airway malformation (CPAM). Cases of malignant transformation of CPAM may have represented a misdiagnosis of PPB. Patients are younger at diagnosis and have a much better prognosis than patients with the other types.

  ▪ Type II—Cystic and solid

  ▪ Type III—Purely solid

Next steps in management

Biopsy is necessary to confirm the diagnosis. Surgery is the mainstay of therapy. Chemotherapy is also indicated.

Further reading

1. Naffaa LN, Donnelly LF. Imaging findings in pleuropulmonary blastoma. Pediatr Radiol. 2005 Apr;35(4):387–391.
2. Orazi C. Inserra A, Schingo PM, et al. Pleuropulmonary blastoma, a distinctive neoplasm of childhood: report of three cases. Pediatr Radiol. 2007 Apr;37(4):337–344.

History

▶ 3-day-old 36-week-gestation baby with respiratory distress.

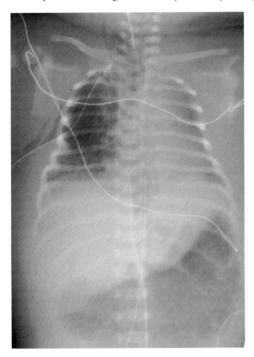

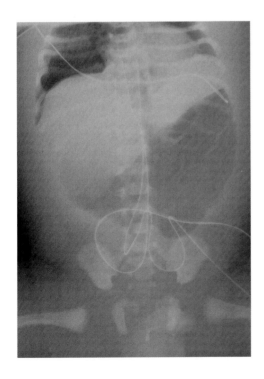

Case 120   Air Leak Phenomena

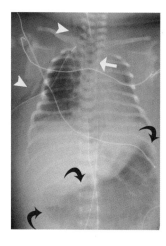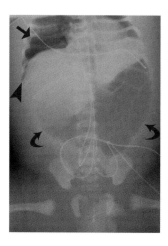

Findings

▶ AP radiograph of the chest (left) shows a high endotracheal tube, umbilical catheters, and a right chest tube. There is air overlying the superior mediastinum (arrow) and in the subcutaneous tissues of the neck and chest wall (arrowheads), and free intraperitoneal air (curved arrows). Note also body wall edema, which is a sign of poor clinical status.

▶ Radiograph of the abdomen obtained later the same day shows air at the right lung base (arrow) with a sharp border of the right hemidiaphragm and heart compared to the left and deep sulcus sign (arrowhead), indicating pneumothorax in a supine patient. Free intraperitoneal air is seen diffusely (curved arrows).

Differential diagnosis

Pneumothorax may accumulate medially in a supine neonate and can mimic pneumomediastinum. Pneumomediastinum occurs in the midline and elevates the lobes of the thymus outward ("angel wing" or "batwing" sign) and outlines the superior margin of the heart, while pneumothorax compresses the thymus against the mediastinum.

Teaching points

▶ Air leak phenomena complicate positive-pressure ventilation therapy in neonates as well as adults, but the findings may be more difficult to discern in neonates. Sick premature neonates are very labile and are nearly always imaged supine. The lungs affected with surfactant deficiency or pneumonia are noncompliant and may not collapse despite the presence of a relatively large pneumothorax.

▶ Mediastinal air may track into the retroperitoneum or peritoneal cavity through diaphragmatic foramina.

▶ In pneumopericardium, air surrounds the heart but does not extend above the origin of the great vessels or displace the thymus. Unlike pneumomediastinum, pneumopericardium must be decompressed urgently to prevent cardiac tamponade.

Next steps in management

Pneumothorax is treated with needle or tube decompression. Oscillating ventilators can be used to decrease airway pressures while maintaining oxygenation.

Further reading

1. Newman B. Imaging of medical disease of the newborn lung. Radiol Clin North Am. 1999 Nov;36(6):1049–1065.
2. Agrons GA, Courtney SE, Stocker JT, Markowitz RI. From the archives of the AFIP: Lung disease in premature neonates: radiologic-pathologic correlation. Radiographics. 2005 Jul–Aug;25(4):1047–1073.

History

▶ 2-day-old 26-week premature infant with respiratory distress. The second image is 1 day later.

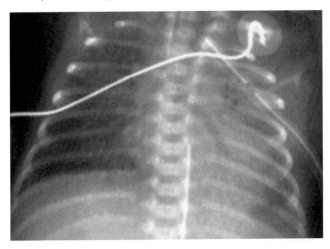

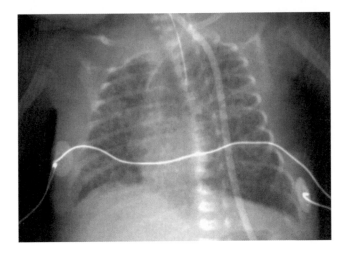

Case 121 Surfactant Deficiency Disease (SDD) Complicated by Pulmonary Interstitial Emphysema (PIE)

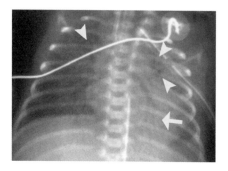 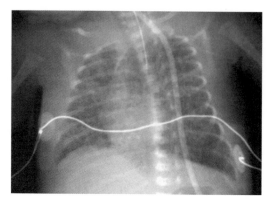

Findings

▶ Initial AP radiograph (left) demonstrates low lung volumes and diffuse granular opacities with branching, tapering air bronchograms (arrow), consistent with surfactant deficiency. Additionally, there are tubular and cystic lucencies (arrowheads) near the hila, which are not branching and tapering, indicating early PIE.

▶ Subsequent AP radiograph (right) shows bilateral diffuse cystic lucencies and increased lung volumes consistent with progression of PIE.

Differential diagnosis

Late changes mimic chronic lung disease, but the rate of progression to this appearance is much faster in PIE.

Teaching points

▶ SDD, previously known as hyaline membrane disease, is the condition in infants born at 34 weeks gestation or less resulting from immaturity of the lungs and lack of surfactant production by type II pneumocytes. Surfactant decreases the surface tension in the walls of the alveoli, allowing them to remain open in exhalation and decreasing the work of breathing.

▶ Therapy includes oxygen, positive-pressure ventilation, and exogenous surfactant. Surfactant causes marked, although sometimes patchy, clearing of the lungs within 24 to 48 hours. A sudden diffuse increase in opacity suggests a complication such as left-to-right shunting through a patent ductus arteriosus or pulmonary hemorrhage.

▶ With positive-pressure ventilation of noncompliant lungs, the alveoli may rupture and air can dissect into the interlobular septa and lymphatics, causing the findings above. If the patient survives, PIE air collections may coalesce to form large pseudocysts called persistent pulmonary interstitial emphysema. On CT, the air collections contain lines and dots (bronchovascular bundles).

Next steps in management

PIE is treated with high-frequency, oscillating ventilators that produce good oxygenation with decreased airway pressures.

Further reading

1. Newman B. Imaging of medical disease of the newborn lung. Radiol Clin North Am. 1999 Nov;36(6):1049–1065.
2. Donnelly LF, Lucaya J, Ozelame V, et al. CT findings and temporal course of persistent pulmonary interstitial emphysema: a multiinstitutional study. AJR Am J Roentgenology. 2003;180:1129–1133.

History

▶ 4-week-old 26-week premature infant with persistent ventilator requirement.

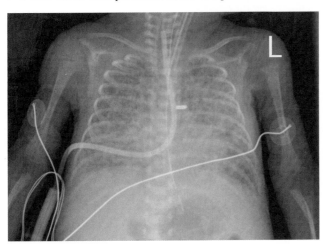

Case 122   Chronic Lung Disease of Prematurity

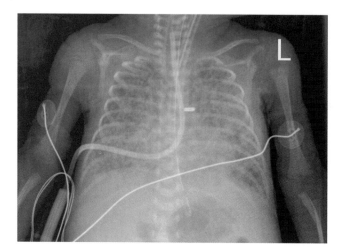

Findings

▶ AP radiograph shows diffuse coarse interstitial markings and small cystic changes with mildly increased lung volumes. Also note patent ductus arteriosus (PDA) clip.

Differential diagnosis

The diffuse cystic changes of chronic lung disease are similar to those of pulmonary interstitial emphysema.

Teaching points

▶ Chronic lung disease, previously known as bronchopulmonary dysplasia, is a complication of oxygen and positive-pressure ventilation therapy, usually for surfactant deficiency. The condition is defined clinically as a persistent oxygen requirement after 28 days of life. The use of exogenous surfactant decreases the risk of progression to chronic lung disease.

▶ Early in surfactant deficiency disease, radiographs show diffuse granular opacities, air bronchograms, and low lung volumes (prior to ventilator treatment). Over the next few days, there may be patchy or complete clearing of opacities after exogenous surfactant. Persistent opacities become coarser and cystic changes develop beginning in the second week in infants who develop chronic lung disease.

▶ The subsequent course usually consists of recurrent episodes of atelectasis and pulmonary edema, which are evident on follow-up radiographs. Comparison prior exams are helpful.

▶ The changes of chronic lung disease develop somewhat slowly. Development of bilateral white-out of the lungs at the end of the first week of life suggests left-to-right shunting has developed through a PDA. In the fetus, pulmonary pressures are high, as blood is not oxygenated in the lungs. This pressure normally decreases after birth but remains elevated in neonates with lung disease. As the lung disease improves, the pulmonary pressure decreases. When systemic pressure exceeds pulmonary arterial pressure, the blood flow shunts through the PDA from left to right.

Next steps in management

The treatment is mainly supportive.

Further reading

1. Newman B. Imaging of medical disease of the newborn lung. Radiol Clin North Am. 1999 Nov;36(6):1049–1065.
2. Agrons GA, Courtney SE, Stocker JT, Markowitz RI. From the archives of the AFIP: Lung disease in premature neonates: radiologic-pathologic correlation. Radiographics. 2005 Jul–Aug;25(4):1047–1073.

History

► Newborn with respiratory distress.

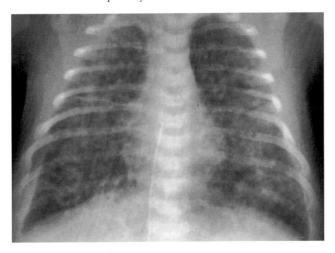

Case 123 Meconium Aspiration

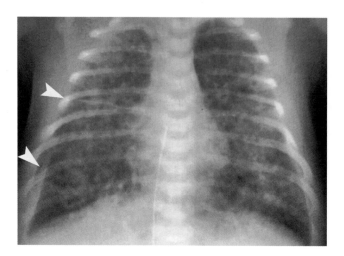

Findings

▶ AP radiograph demonstrates hyperinflated lungs, coarse increased markings, and right pleural fluid (arrowheads).

Differential diagnosis

Bilateral symmetric findings suggest medical lung disease as opposed to surgical entities such as diaphragmatic hernia or congenital lung malformation. The differential diagnosis depends on whether the infant is term or preterm. For a preterm infant, the diagnosis is usually surfactant deficiency disease. For a term infant, the differential diagnosis includes transient tachypnea of the newborn (TTN) and neonatal pneumonia. TTN causes mild to moderate respiratory distress and resolves within 48 to 72 hours. Predisposing factors include cesarean section and precipitous delivery in which there is no thoracic squeeze to expel fetal lung fluid. Findings of hyperinflation and coarse markings favor meconium aspiration.

Teaching points

▶ Aspiration of thick meconium causes obstruction of small and medium airways, leading to air trapping and atelectasis. Meconium also causes a chemical pneumonitis.

▶ Radiographs show hyperinflation and alternating foci of atelectasis and air trapping. Pleural effusion and air leak complications are common.

▶ Meconium aspiration is a leading cause of persistent pulmonary hypertension. Hypoxemia causes pulmonary arterial pressures to remain high as in fetal life. Right-to-left shunting occurs across a patent ductus arteriosus, leading to more hypoxemia. Therapy may include inhaled nitric oxide, which is a potent vasodilator. In severe cases, extracorporeal membrane oxygenation (ECMO) may be required. Cannulas are placed in the jugular vein and the carotid artery, and blood is circulated through a semipermeable membrane across which gas exchange occurs. ECMO therapy requires anticoagulation, and intracranial hemorrhage is a contraindication to ECMO.

Next steps in management

Survival of infants with meconium aspiration is much improved since the advent of ECMO.

Further reading

1. Newman B. Imaging of medical disease of the newborn lung. Radiol Clin North Am. 1999 Nov;36(6):1049–1065.
2. Barnacle AM, Smith LC, Hiorns MP. The role of imaging during ECMO in pediatric respiratory failure. AJR Am J Roentgenol. 2006 Jan;186(1):58–66.

History

▶ 3-year-old boy with wheeze.

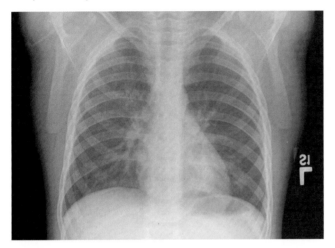

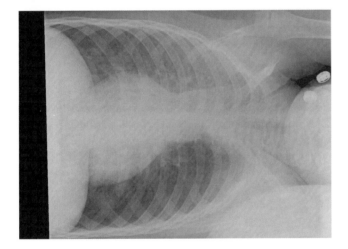

Case 124 Left Mainstem Bronchus Aspirated Foreign Body

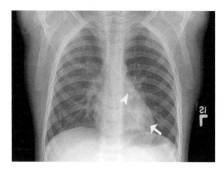 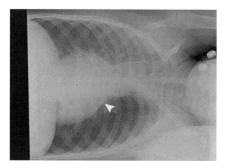

Findings

▶ PA chest radiograph (left) demonstrates slight hyperlucency of the left lung compared to the right, left retrocardiac opacity representing atelectasis (arrow), and a density over the left mainstem bronchus (arrowhead).

▶ Left lateral decubitus view of the chest (right) shows the same density in the left hilum (arrowhead) and failure of the left lung to collapse with decubitus positioning.

Differential diagnosis

The retrocardiac opacity could also represent pneumonia in a febrile child, but that diagnosis would not explain the air trapping. Air trapping and atelectasis are signs of airway obstruction. In adults, lung cancer is a common endobronchial lesion. In young children, aspirated foreign body is most likely.

Teaching points

▶ Aspiration of a foreign body may present as a dramatic event or with indolent symptoms related to chronic airway obstruction. It is important to maintain a high index of suspicion in crawling infants.

▶ Generally, airway foreign bodies are not radiopaque. The radiographic findings are due to airway obstruction. The airways are larger in inhalation than in exhalation, especially in children who have pliable airways. The foreign object acts as a check valve, causing air trapping as well as atelectasis. Air trapping is difficult to detect on inspiratory examinations and routine radiographs may be normal despite the presence of a foreign body. Exhalation can be induced with decubitus positioning of the chest. The dependent lung normally collapses. Failure to collapse is usually due to an aspirated foreign body. CT virtual bronchoscopy may be useful in localizing foreign bodies.

▶ Aspirated foreign body should be suspected in young children with pneumonia that recurs or fails to clear or with air leak phenomena.

Next steps in management

Acute airway foreign bodies are removed with bronchoscopic guidance. Chronic foreign bodies resulting in bronchiectasis usually require lobectomy.

Further reading

1. Lee KS, Boiselle PM. Update on multidetector computed tomography imaging of the airways. J Thoracic Imaging. 2010 May;25(2):112–124.
2. Yedururi S, Gillerman RP, Chung T, et al. Multimodality imaging of tracheobronchial disorders in children. Radiographics. 2008 May–June;28(3):e29.

Part 7   Musculoskeletal System

History

▶ Prenatal ultrasound image of the femur and postmortem radiograph of the infant.

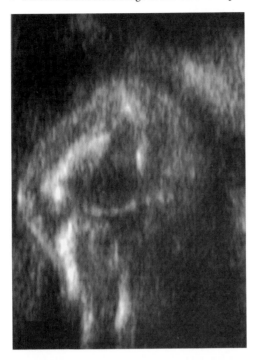

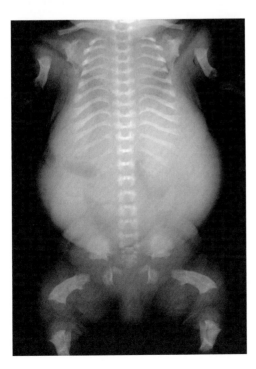

Case 125 Thanatophoric Dysplasia

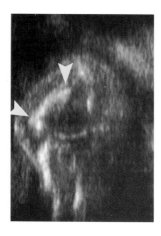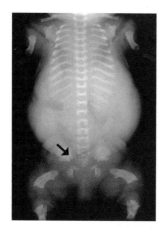

Findings

▶ Coronal sonographic image of the femur (left) shows a curved appearance similar to a telephone receiver (arrowheads).

▶ Postmortem AP radiograph of the infant (right) shows handle-bar clavicles, symmetrically short ribs and a small thorax, platyspondyly with H-, U-, and inverted-U-shaped vertebral bodies, small flared iliac wings, flat acetabular roofs, narrow sacrosciatic notches (arrow), and "telephone-receiver" femora.

Differential diagnosis

Other lethal skeletal dysplasias include asphyxiating thoracic dysplasia (Jeune syndrome), which also demonstrates short ribs and a small thorax with pulmonary hypoplasia. The finding of platyspondyly helps to distinguish thanatophoric dysplasia from Jeune syndrome.

Teaching points

▶ Thanatophoric dysplasia is part of the achondroplasia group of skeletal dysplasias, which share abnormalities of the same gene product, fibroblast growth factor receptor 3. Thanatophoric dysplasia is probably the most common lethal bone dysplasia.

▶ The poor prognosis is due to the short ribs and very small thorax, which cause secondary pulmonary hypoplasia. Prenatal ultrasound features include a thoracic circumference at the level of the four-chamber view of the heart that is less than 80% of the abdominal circumference at the level of the portal vein. Also, on axial images, the ribs extend less than two thirds of the way around the circumference of the chest.

▶ Some patients also have kleeblattschädel, or clover-leaf skull, which is a deformity that results from premature closure of all cranial sutures so that growth can occur only through bowing of the membranous portions of the skull.

▶ The appearance of the pelvis is common to many skeletal dysplasias, but the telephone-receiver appearance of the femora and humeri is specific for thanatophoric dysplasia.

Next steps in management

Thanatophoric dysplasia is almost invariably lethal.

Further reading

1. Lemyre E, Azouz EM, Teebi AS, et al. Bone dysplasia series. Achondroplasia, hypochondroplasia and thanatophoric dysplasia: review and update. Can Assoc Radiol J. 1999 Jun;50(3):185–197.
2. Cassart M. Suspected fetal skeletal malformations or bone diseases: how to explore. Pediatr Radiol. 2010 Jun;40(6):1046–1051.

History

► 3-year-old with short stature.

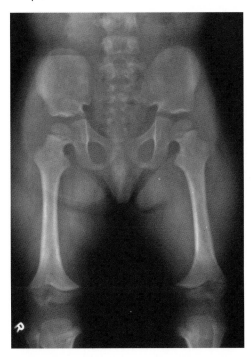

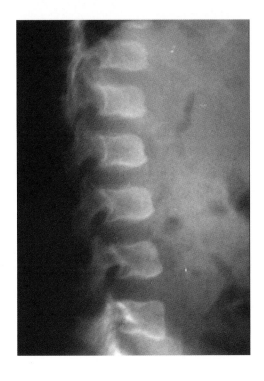

Case 126 Achondroplasia

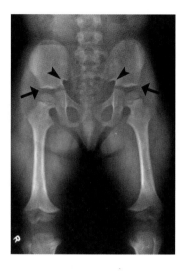 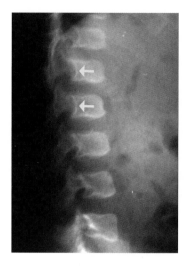

Findings

▶ AP radiograph (left) of the pelvis and upper legs reveals flared iliac wings with flat acetabular roofs (arrows) and narrow sacrosciatic notches (arrowheads). The femora are shortened with wide, flared distal metaphyses with a chevron appearance.

▶ Lateral radiograph of the spine (right) demonstrates short pedicles causing narrowing of the spinal canal. Posterior vertebral scalloping (arrows) is also noted.

Differential diagnosis

Thanatophoric dysplasia also results from an abnormality of the same gene locus, but is lethal due to very short ribs and a small thorax, which cause secondary pulmonary hypoplasia. Other findings of thanatophoric dysplasia include platyspondyly and "telephone-receiver" femora.

Teaching points

▶ Achondroplasia, the most common non-lethal skeletal dysplasia, results from an autosomal dominant defect involving fibroblast growth factor receptor 3, which is important in enchondral bone formation.

▶ The clinically apparent frontal bossing is due to midface (enchondral bone formation) hypoplasia with normal skull growth (membranous bone formation). The skull base is also affected, so that the foramen magnum and neural foramina are small, which may result in neurologic consequences.

▶ The distance between the pedicles of the lumbar spine decreases from craniad to caudad, which is the opposite of the normal progression. The short pedicles cause congenital spinal canal stenosis. Degenerative disk disease may cause paraplegia in adulthood. Exaggerated lumbar lordosis is frequent.

▶ Limb shortening is primarily rhizomelic (proximal), but all bones of the extremities are shortened. The hands demonstrate brachydactyly and metaphyseal cupping.

Next steps in management

Skeletal deformities may be treated individually with surgical procedures.

Further reading

1. Lachman RS. Neurologic abnormalities in the skeletal dysplasias: a clinical and radiological perspective. Am J Med Genet. 1997 Mar 3;69(1):33–43.
2. Cheema JI, Grissom LE, Harcke HT. Radiographic characteristics of lower-extremity bowing in children. Radiographics. 2003 Jul–Aug;23(4):871–880.

History

▶ 8-month-old, rule out bilateral clavicular fractures.

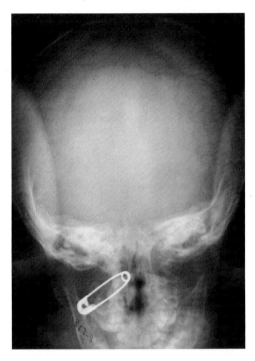

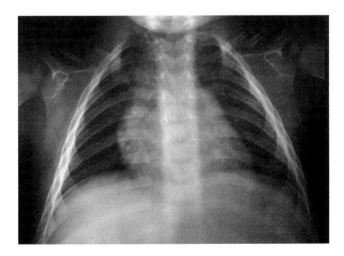

Case 127 Cleidocranial Dysplasia

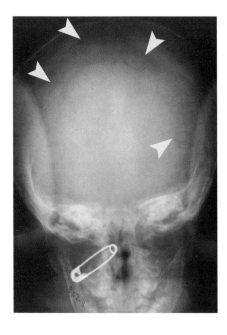
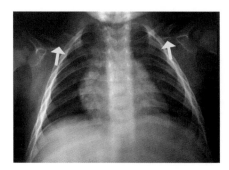

Findings

► Towne view of the skull (left) shows multiple intrasutural or wormian bones (arrowheads).
► PA radiograph of the chest (right) shows bilateral small clavicles with pseudarthroses (arrows), downward-sloping ribs, and a triangular configuration to the thorax.

Differential diagnosis

The differential diagnosis for wormian bones includes normal (8–10 small intrasutural bones), osteogenesis imperfecta, hypothyroidism, pyknodysostosis, Menke's kinky hair syndrome, and hypophosphatasia.

Teaching points

► Cleidocranial dysplasia is an autosomal dominant condition that affects membranous bone development. Short stature is mild.
► The anterior fontanelle may be quite wide. The clavicles are absent or hypoplastic. The symphysis pubis is wide due to absence or hypoplasia of the pubic bones. The iliac wings are narrow. The distal phalanges are tapered.

Next steps in management

Genetic counseling is helpful. Dental treatment is necessary for supernumerary teeth.

Further reading

1. Markowitz RI, Zackai E. A pragmatic approach to the radiologic diagnosis of pediatric syndromes and skeletal dysplasias. Radiol Clin North Am. 2001 Jul;39(4):791–802, xi.
2. Gupta SK, Sharma OP, Malhotra S, Gupta S. Cleido-cranial dysostosis—skeletal abnormalities. Australas Radiol. 1992 Aug;36(3):238–242.

History

▶ 5-year-old with multiple deformities.

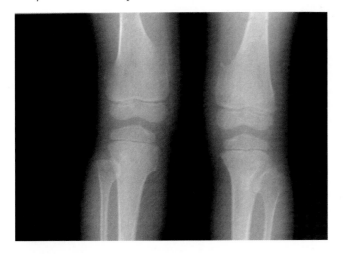

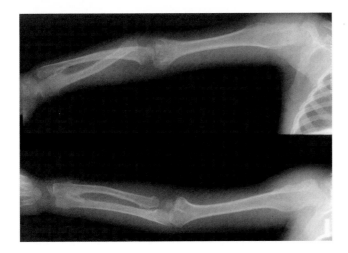

Case 128   Multiple Hereditary Exostoses (MHE)

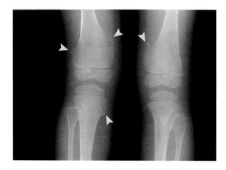 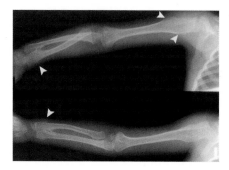

Findings

▸ Radiographs of the knees and right upper extremity show multiple sessile and pedunculated excrescences (arrowheads) directed away from the physis. The cortex and medullary cavity of these are continuous with those of the adjacent bone. These cause widening and deformity of the metadiaphyses of the involved bones. Note that the ulna is shortened and the distal radius is bowed (pseudo-Madelung deformity).

Differential diagnosis

Common generalized deforming bone diseases include Ollier disease and polyostotic fibrous dysplasia.

Teaching points

▸ MHE is an autosomal dominant condition of multiple osteochondromas. Osteochondromas represent one of the most common dysplasias of bones. Most commonly, these involve long bones, particularly around the knee, the ribs, and the pelvis, but they can arise in any bone with a physis. MHE generally presents by age 10 years.

▸ Complications include pain, deformity, fracture, local neurovascular compromise, and sarcomatous degeneration. The last is very rare in solitary osteochondromas, even if they are induced by radiation therapy, but the incidence in MHE is about 5%, generally occurring in adulthood.

▸ Findings suggesting malignant degeneration are increased pain, growth after skeletal maturity, increased thickness of the cartilage cap seen on MR or CT, erosion of the cortex, new increased lucency in the lesion, or soft-tissue mass.

▸ MR is superior for the evaluation of the cartilage cap, which is bright on T2-weighted images. Fat-suppressed images distinguish the cartilage cap from fatty bone marrow. A cartilage cap less than 1 cm in thickness is definitely benign. A cap of greater than 2 cm indicates malignant degeneration.

Next steps in management

Surgical resection is performed to treat pain, deformity, and neurovascular complications. Patients are followed with radiographs.

Further reading

1. Murphey MD, Choi JJ, Kransdorf MS, et al. Imaging of osteochondroma: variants and complications with radiologic-patho-logic correlation. Radiographics 2000;20:1407–1434.
2. Vanhoenacker FM, Van Hul W, Wuyts W, et al. Hereditary multiple exostoses: from genetics to clinical syndrome and com-plications. Eur J Radiol. 2001;40:208–217.

History

▶ Boy with worsening hand deformities. First image is at age 10 years and second at 18 years.

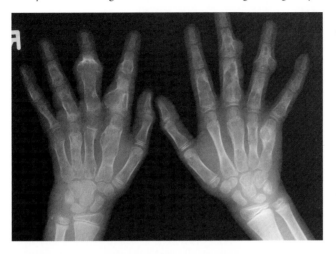

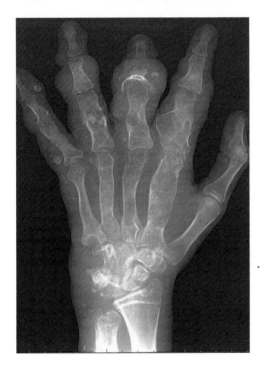

Case 129   Maffucci Syndrome (Enchondromatosis with Venous Malformations)

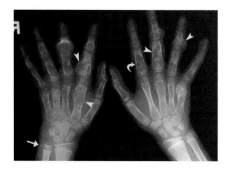 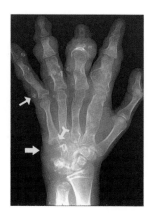

Findings

▶ Radiograph of the hands at age 10 years (left) shows multiple expansile lucent lesions surrounded by a thin rim of cortex (arrowheads). Less expansile lesions show endosteal scalloping (curved arrow). A single soft-tissue calcification is visible (arrow).

▶ By age 18, the lesions have grown larger and more soft-tissue pleboliths are visible (arrow). A soft-tissue mass (block arrow) causing indolent bone erosion (tailed arrow) likely represents a vascular malformation.

Differential diagnosis

Common generalized deforming bone diseases also include multiple hereditary exostoses and polyostotic fibrous dysplasia.

Teaching points

▶ Enchondromatosis, or Ollier disease, is a nonhereditary mesodermal dysplasia with multiple cartilaginous lesions of short tubular bones and the metadiaphyses of long bones, resulting from abnormal enchondral ossification at the physis. The small bones of the hands are most often affected.

▶ Maffucci syndrome is characterized by multiple enchondromas and vascular malformations, usually venous.

▶ Radiographs of lesions involving long bones may demonstrate arc-and-whorl-pattern calcifications. Periosteal reaction is absent.

▶ At MR imaging, the signal intensity of the lesions follows that of cartilage on all sequences. On T1-weighted images the lesions are isointense to muscle. T2-weighted sequences reveal predominantly hyperintense signal. Adjacent bone marrow edema and enhancement are absent.

▶ Solitary enchondromas rarely undergo malignant transformation, but the lesions in patients with Ollier disease or Maffucci syndrome do have a significant risk of transformation to chondrosarcoma in adulthood. Signs of malignant transformation include erosion of adjacent bone and development of a soft-tissue mass.

Next steps in management

Surgical resection is performed for symptomatic lesions. Patients are followed with radiographs.

Further reading

1. Robbins MR, Murphey MD. Imaging of osteochondroma: variants and complications with radiologic-pathologic correlation. Semin Musculoskelet Radiol. 2000;4:45–58.
2. Brien EW, Mirra JM, Kerr R. Benign and malignant cartilage tumors of bone and joint: their anatomic and theoretical basis with emphasis on radiology, pathology and clinical biology. I. The intramedullary cartilage tumors. Skeletal Radiol. 1997;26:325–353.

History

▸ 13-year-old girl with left hip pain and limp.

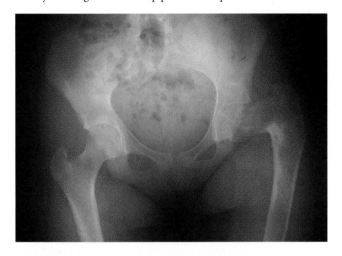

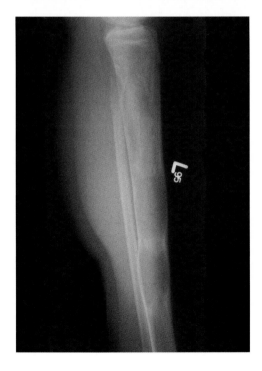

Case 130 Polyostotic Fibrous Dysplasia

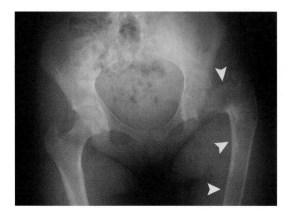 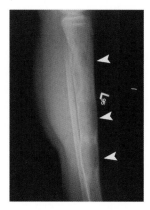

Findings

▶ AP radiograph of the pelvis (left) reveals that the medullary cavity of the metaphysis and diaphysis of the left femur is diffusely abnormal and slightly expanded with ground-glass-opacity material (arrowheads) causing endosteal scalloping. Acute varus bowing of the proximal femur represents the "shepherd's crook" deformity.

▶ Lateral radiograph of the left tibia (right) shows similar findings (arrowheads).

Differential diagnosis

For solitary lesions, non-ossifying fibroma and solitary bone cyst should be considered. For multiple lesions, consider enchondromatosis, which also causes lucent lesions but predominantly in the hands. Additionally, enchondromas of long bones often demonstrate the arc-and-whorl calcifications of the cartilaginous matrix.

Teaching points

▶ Fibrous dysplasia is a developmental abnormality of osteoblast maturation in which the marrow space is replaced by immature fibro-osseous tissue. Most cases are monostotic. Polyostotic fibrous dysplasia is more common in girls and frequently predominates on one side of the body. McCune-Albright syndrome consists of polyostotic fibrous dysplasia with precocious puberty and Coast-of-Maine café-au-lait spots. Monostotic lesions present in adolescents and young adults, while polyostotic disease is typically manifest by age 10 years.

▶ Fibrous dysplasia may affect any bone but most commonly involves long bones, especially the proximal femur and tibia, the ribs, and the craniofacial bones.

▶ Lesions arise centrally or eccentrically in the metaphysis and diaphysis of long bones and do not cross the unfused physis. The opacity depends on the relative content of fibrous and osseous components, ranging from ground-glass to radiolucent.

▶ MR signal intensity is variable on T2-weighted sequences depending on the composition of osseous (hyperintense) versus fibrous (hypointense) matrix. Lesions are isointense to muscle on T1-weighted images.

▶ Risk of malignant transformation to osteo- or fibrosarcoma is low but higher in polyostotic or radiation-induced lesions.

Next steps in management

Surgery is performed as necessary to treat deformity.

Further reading

1. Fitzpatrick KA, Taljanovic MS, Speer DP, et al Imaging findings of fibrous dysplasia with histopathologic and intraoperative correlation. AJR Am J Roentgenol. 2004;182:1389–1398.
2. Kransdorf MJ, Moser RP Jr, Gilkey FW. Fibrous dysplasia. Radiographics 1990;10:519–537.

History

▸ 15-month-old girl with limb deformity.

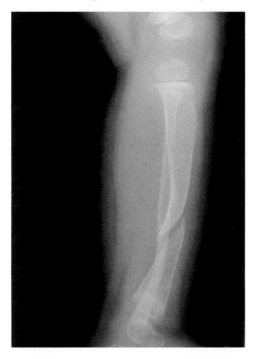

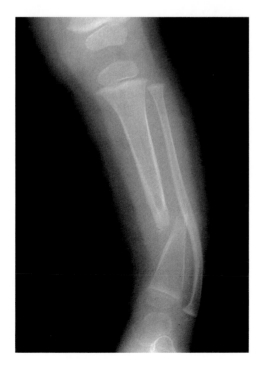

Case 131 Tibial Pseudarthrosis in Neurofibromatosis Type 1 (NF1)

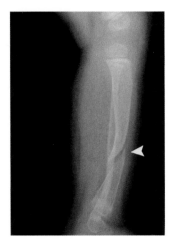 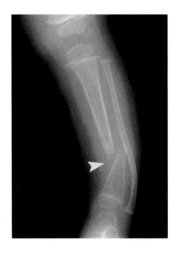

Findings

▶ Lateral and AP radiographs of the lower leg reveal discontinuity of the mid-portion of the tibia with well-corticated edges consistent with pseudarthrosis (arrowheads). There is anterolateral angulation of the tibia and anterolateral bowing of the fibula.

Differential diagnosis

Congenital tibial bowing that is not associated with NF1 is posteromedial.

Teaching points

▶ NF1, or von Recklinghausen disease, is the most common phakomatosis. The disease is caused by an autosomal dominant gene mutation on chromosome 17 that results in loss of a negative regulator of the RAS proto-oncogene, cellular overgrowth, and tumor formation.

▶ Musculoskeletal manifestations may be due to erosion by tumors (neurofibromas), dural ectasia, or mesodermal dysplasia.

▶ Long-bone pseudarthrosis may involve the tibia, femur, radius, ulna, or humerus and is usually unilateral. Generally, the pseudarthrosis is not truly congenital, but mesodermal dysplasia caused a bowing deformity that fractures and does not heal.

▶ Spinal manifestations include pedicle hypoplasia, scoliosis with or without vertebral body dysplasia, posterior vertebral body scalloping (due to dural ectasia or neurofibromas), and neural foraminal widening by neurofibromas.

▶ Ribs may be ribbon-like due to neurofibromas of the intercostal nerves or to mesodermal dysplasia.

▶ Other skeletal findings may include sphenoid wing hypoplasia and multiple non-ossifying fibromas.

Next steps in management

If found in a patient without a known diagnosis of NF1, other stigmata should be sought with skin examination and MR of the brain, as 70% of patients with anterolateral tibial bowing/pseudarthrosis have NF1. The pseudarthrosis may be treated with osteotomy and fusion, but often recurs.

Further reading

1. Crawford AH, Schorry EK. Neurofibromatosis update. J Pediatr Orthop. 2006;26:413–423.
2. Rossi SE, Erasmus JJ, McAdams HP, et al. Thoracic manifestations of neurofibromatosis 1. AJR Am J Roentgenol 1999;173:1631–1638.

History

▶ Newborn with respiratory distress.

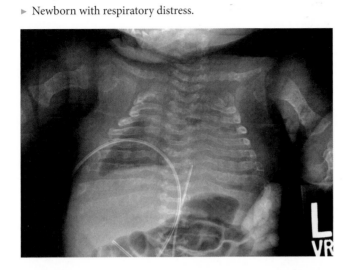

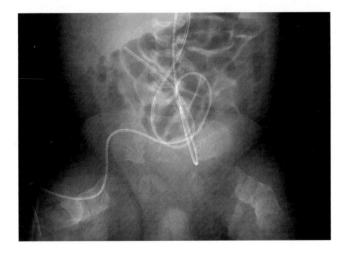

Case 132   Osteogenesis Imperfecta (OI) Type II

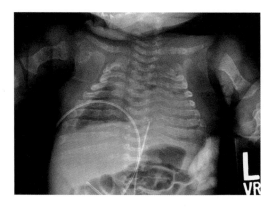 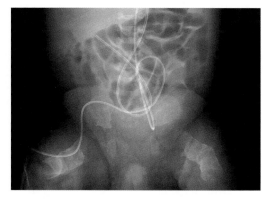

Findings

▶ Plain radiographs reveal diffuse osteopenia, collapsed vertebral bodies, small thorax with beaded ribs, and short, widened, and crumpled long bones with thin cortices (accordion femora).

Differential diagnosis

The osteopenia and bowing deformities suggest OI type II. The skull would show absent or poor ossification. Lethal skeletal dysplasias also include thanatophoric dysplasia and asphyxiating thoracic dysplasia. Both have short but not beaded ribs. Thanatophoric dysplasia is distinguished by true platyspondyly and telephone-receiver femora. Kleeblattschädel is seen in some patients with thanatophoric dysplasia. Asphyxiating thoracic dysplasia is distinguished by a normal spine and cone-shaped epiphyses. For older infants with other types of OI, the main differential consideration is inflicted trauma. Inflicted trauma in young infants usually involves fractures of the metaphysis rather than diaphysis and absence of the osteoporosis, cortical thinning, blue sclera, and wormian bones characteristic of OI. The hypothesized existence of so-called "temporary brittle bone disease" been examined in several reviews that are highly critical of the methodology used to support it.

Teaching points

▶ Four types are recognized:
  ▪ Type I—mild osteopenia with normal stature and wormian bones (greater than 8–10). Some have blue sclera with normal teeth while others have normal sclera with dentinogenesis imperfecta (DI). Repeated fractures heal with exuberant callus and lead to bowing deformities.
  ▪ Type II—usually diagnosed in the second trimester on ultrasound with femur length greater than 3 standard deviations below the mean for gestational age. The sclerae are always blue.
  ▪ Type III—perinatal presentation with blue-gray sclera that later become white, DI, wormian bones, severe osteoporosis, and early and recurrent fractures leading to deformity. Bones become shortened, thin, and bowed with very thin cortices.
  ▪ Type IV—similar to type II but with normal sclera and no wormian bones.

Next steps in management

OI type II is invariably lethal.

Further reading

1. Lachman RS. Fetal imaging in the skeletal dysplasias: overview and experience. Pediatr Radiol. 1994;24:413.
2. Mendelson KL. Critical review of "temporary brittle bone disease." Pediatr Radiol. 2005 Oct;35(10):1036–1040.

History

▶ 13-month-old boy with lower limb deformity.

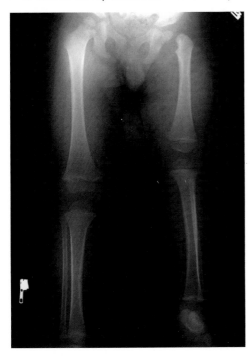

Case 133 Proximal Focal Femoral Deficiency (PFFD)

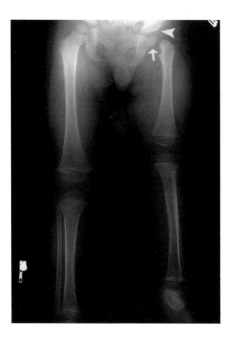

Findings

▶ Scanogram shows shortening of the femur with apparent dissociation of the femoral head epiphysis (arrow) and the femoral neck as the cartilaginous connection is not radiographically apparent. Note also the shallow acetabulum (arrowhead).

Teaching points

▶ PFFD is a spectrum of developmental abnormalities of the femur ranging from mild shortening to severe predominantly proximal deficiency and acetabular dysplasia.

▶ Most cases are sporadic. Other ipsilateral deformities may be present, including fibular hemimelia.

▶ In infants the femoral head and/or its connection to the rest of the femur may be formed of cartilage and invisible on radiographs, as in this case. The finding of a well-formed acetabulum indicates the presence of a femoral head. The cartilaginous head and/or connection to the femoral diaphysis may be visualized with ultrasound or MRI. MRI is particularly helpful for defining the anatomy, including cartilaginous portions of the bones, ligaments, and surrounding muscles, which are often hypoplastic.

▶ Acetabular deficiency is present even in mild cases, and unlike developmental dysplasia of the hip, in which there is anterior deficiency, in PFFD the deficiency is posterior.

Next steps in management

Preoperative MRI is very helpful. The aim of surgery is often to make the limb a better attachment for a prosthesis. Rotationplasty of the tibia entails turning the foot so that the toes point posteriorly and the ankle can be used as a knee.

Further reading

1. Bernaerts A, Pouillon M, De Ridder K, Vanhoenacker F. Value of magnetic resonance imaging in early assessment of proximal focal femoral deficiency (PFFD). JBR-BTR. 2006 Nov–Dec;89(6):325–327.
2. Anton CG, Applegate KE, Kuivila TE, Wilkes DC. Proximal femoral focal deficiency (PFFD): more than an abnormal hip. Semin Musculoskelet Radiol. 1999;3(3):215–226.

History

▶ 10-year-old boy with wrist pain.

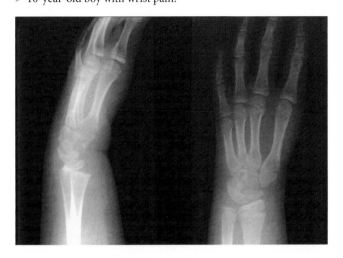

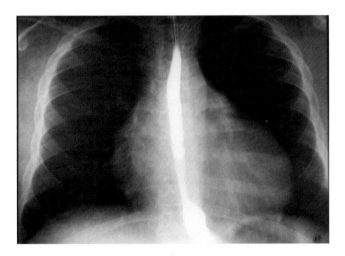

Case 134 Radial Ray Anomaly in Holt-Oram Syndrome

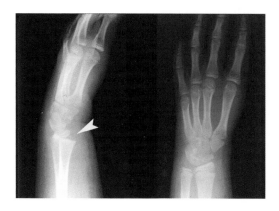
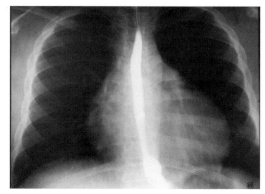

Findings

▸ AP radiograph of the upper extremity (left) reveals a Salter-Harris II fracture of the distal radius (arrowhead) and complete absence of the first ray.

▸ Chest radiograph shows enlargement of the heart due to ventricular septal defect.

Differential diagnosis

Radial ray anomalies are often unilateral and sporadic, but, if bilateral, they are likely to be associated with one of several conditions, including VACTERL association, Holt-Oram syndrome, Fanconi anemia, thrombo-cytopenia-absent radius (TAR) syndrome, Cornelia de Lange syndrome, valproic acid exposure, and trisomies 13 and 18. TAR is distinguished from the others by the presence of the thumb. TAR and Fanconi anemia are associated with abnormal blood counts. Holt-Oram syndrome, Fanconi anemia, and VACTERL are associated with congenital heart disease. For Holt-Oram patients, the most common cardiac defects are atrial or ventricular septal defect.

Teaching points

▸ Radial ray anomalies range from hypoplasia of the thumb to complete absence of the radius.

▸ When the radius is completely absent, there is radial and volar deviation of the hand causing a "club hand" appearance. The forearm is short and the ulna may be curved and thick. If there is a remnant of the radius it may be fused to the ulna. The radial carpal bones may be deformed or absent.

▸ Half of cases are bilateral.

Next steps in management

Children with radial ray anomalies should be screened for associated conditions with renal ultrasound, echocardiography, and complete blood count. Treatment is serial casting or splinting. Thumb reconstruction or pollicization of the index finger may be performed.

Further reading

1. Maschke SD, Seitz W, Lawton J. Radial longitudinal deficiency. J Am Acad Orthop Surg. 2007 Jan;15(1):41–52.
2. Kennelly MM, Moran P. A clinical algorithm of prenatal diagnosis of radial ray defects with two- and three-dimensional ultrasound. Prenat Diagn. 2007 Aug;27(8):730–737.

History

► 3-month-old with foot deformity.

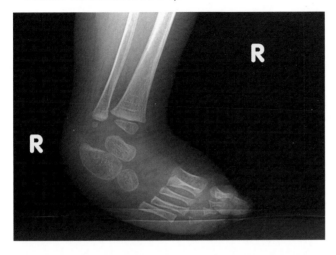

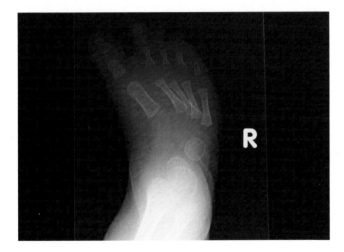

Case 135   Talipes Equinovarus (Clubfoot)

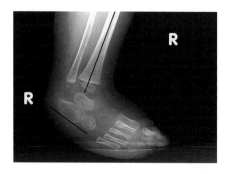 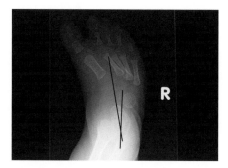

Findings

▶ Lateral (left) and dorsoplantar (DP) radiographs show hindfoot equinus and varus and forefoot varus and supination.

Differential diagnosis

Congenital vertical talus and skewfoot.

Teaching points

▶ Risk factors include family history, abnormal in utero positioning (e.g., oligohydramnios), and decreased fetal leg movement (e.g., spinal dysraphism). There is an association with developmental dysplasia of the hip.

▶ Foot deformities are evaluated in weight-bearing or forced dorsiflexion. Normally, the angle between the long axes of the tibia and calcaneus (tibiocalcaneal angle) is 60 to 90 degrees. In hindfoot equinus, the anterior calcaneus is plantarflexed and the tibiocalcaneal angle is greater than 90 degrees (left image).

▶ Normally, the angle between the long axes of the talus and calcaneus (talocalcaneal [TC] angle) is 15 to 40 degrees on the DP view and 25 to 45 degrees on the lateral view. In hindfoot varus, the talus is assumed to be fixed relative to the tibia and the anterior calcaneus is rotated medially (varus), so the talus and calcaneus are more parallel than normal and the TC angle is decreased (right image).

▶ Normally, a line drawn through the middle of the talus along its long axis (midtalar line) passes just medial to the base of the first metatarsal. In forefoot varus, the forefoot is rotated medially relative to the ankle and the midtalar line passes lateral to the first metatarsal (right image).

▶ Normally, there is mild overlap of the bases of the metatarsals on the DP and lateral views. In forefoot supination, the foot is rolled so that the plantar surface is directed medially and weight is borne on the outside of the foot. On the DP view, there is more overlap of the metatarsals than normal, while on the lateral view, there is less overlap and the metatarsals are aligned in a ladder-like configuration (left image).

Next steps in management

Casting and bracing is the initial therapy, followed by surgery as necessary.

Further reading

1. Mandell GA, Harcke HT, Kumar SJ. Congenital disorders of the extremities. Top Magn Reson Imaging. 1991 Dec;4(1):1–20.
2. Chung EM. Clubfoot imaging. Emedicine. www.emedicine.com

History

▶ 2-year-old with developmental delay and usual facial appearance.

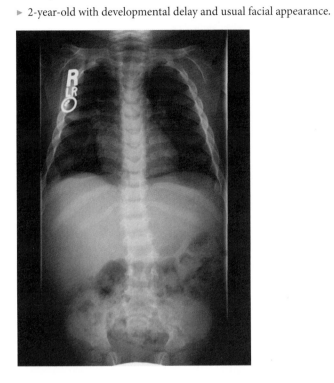

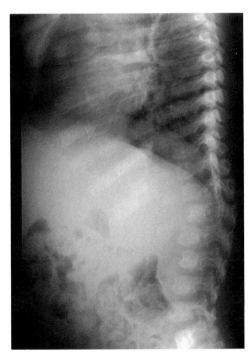

Case 136 Mucopolysaccharidosis Type I (Hurler Syndrome)

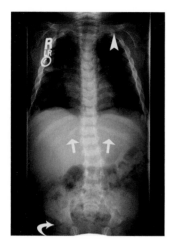 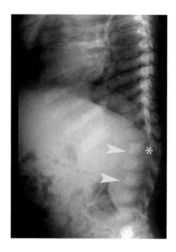

Findings

▶ AP radiograph (left) shows thickened clavicles (arrowhead), oar-shaped lower ribs (arrows), and flared iliac wings with inferior tapering (curved arrow).

▶ Lateral radiograph of the spine reveals focal kyphosis, or gibbus deformity, at the thoracolumbar junction (asterisk) and anteroinferior beaks of the lumbar vertebral bodies (arrowheads).

Differential diagnosis

Other mucopolysaccharidoses and mucolipidoses, including Hunter and Morquio syndromes, cause a similar constellation of radiographic findings termed *dysostosis multiplex*.

Teaching points

▶ Mucopolysaccharidosis type I is an autosomal recessive lysosomal storage disorder resulting from deficiency of the lysosomal enzyme α_1-iduronidase, which is necessary to break down glycosaminoglycans. The result is accumulation of these large molecules within tissues and organs, resulting in multiorgan dysfunction. Hurler syndrome is the most severe form.

▶ Progressive neurodegenerative disease is the clinical hallmark of Hurler disease. Communicating hydrocephalus is common.

▶ Additional radiographic findings include thick calvarium, J-shaped sella turcica, flared iliac wings with inferior tapering and steep acetabular roofs, widened diaphyses, V-shaped carpus, and pointed proximal poles of metacarpals.

▶ Patients with Hurler and Morquio syndrome have an increased incidence of odontoid hypoplasia and atlantoaxial instability.

Next steps in management

Patients are best treated by multidisciplinary teams. Hematopoietic stem cell transplantation and enzyme replacement are new therapies available in the treatment of mucopolysaccharidoses.

Further reading

1. Levin TL, Berdon WE, Lachman RS, et al. Lumbar gibbus in storage diseases and bone dysplasias. Pediatr Radiol. 1997 Apr;27(4):289–294.
2. Scott HS, Bunge S, Gal A, et al. Molecular genetics of mucopolysaccharidosis type I: diagnostic, clinical, and biological implications. Hum Mutat. 1995;6(4):288–302.

History

▶ 18-month-old with limp. Both sides are shown.

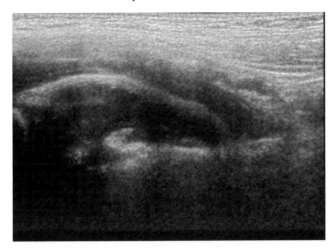

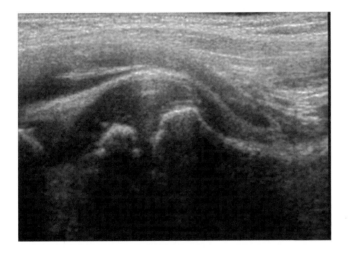

Case 137 Hip Effusion

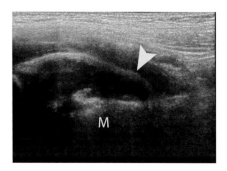
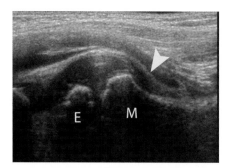

Findings

▶ Longitudinal ultrasound image of the left hip (left) shows a bowed joint capsule (arrowhead) that is separated from the femoral metaphysis (M) by fluid in the joint.

▶ Longitudinal ultrasound image of the asymptomatic right hip (right) shows the normal concave appearance of the joint capsule (arrowhead) that is closely applied to the femoral metaphysis (M). (E = epiphysis)

Differential diagnosis

The most important diagnosis to exclude is septic arthritis. Other causes of hip effusion include toxic (transient) synovitis, inflammatory arthritis, and hemarthrosis due to hemophilia. There is no reliable way to make a definitive diagnosis on the basis of imaging, and joint aspiration is required.

Teaching points

▶ Ultrasound is the most sensitive imaging modality for hip effusion. In contrast to the posterolateral approach that is used in the evaluation of the hip for developmental dysplasia of the hip, the hip is imaged in the parasagittal plane from an anterior approach. Small amounts of fluid accumulate in the anterior recess of the hip before causing lateral joint space widening that can be detected on AP radiographs.

▶ Comparison to the asymptomatic side is helpful. A difference of more than 2 mm in the distance of the joint capsule from the metaphysis is abnormal.

▶ Septic arthritis is most often caused by *Staphylococcus aureus* in children under the age of 2 years and by group B streptococcus or coliform bacteria in older children. Septic arthritis may be due to osteomyelitis, particularly in infants under the age of 18 months, in whom the organisms can cross the physis.

▶ Toxic (transient) synovitis is a self-limited, idiopathic condition that causes pain and a sterile effusion. A history of recent viral illness is common. Toxic synovitis is a diagnosis of exclusion.

Next steps in management

Ultrasound is used to guide hip aspiration. Aspirate lateral to the femoral vessels.

Further reading

1. Bellah R. Ultrasound in pediatric musculoskeletal disease: techniques and applications. Radiol Clin North Am. 2001 Jul;39(4):597–618, ix.
2. Craig JG. Infection: ultrasound-guided procedures. Radiol Clin North Am. 1999;37(4):669–678.

History

▶ 3-year-old with pain and swelling of left ankle. Both ankles are shown.

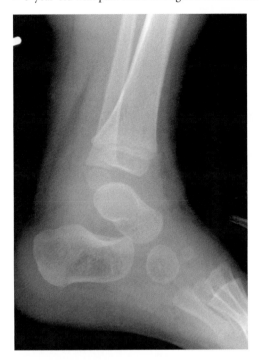

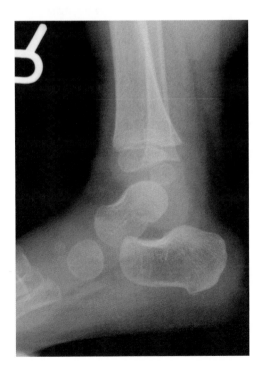

Case 138 Hemophilia A

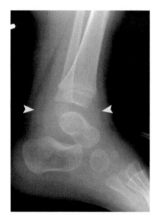 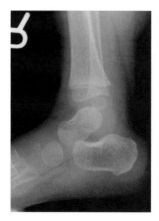

Findings

▶ Lateral radiograph of the left ankle (left) shows a dense effusion (arrowheads), compared to the normal right.

Differential diagnosis

Effusions may be caused by septic joints, toxic synovitis, trauma, and juvenile idiopathic arthritis (JIA). Dense effusion suggests hemarthrosis, such as with hemophilia.

Teaching points

▶ Hemophilia A accounts for the majority of cases and is due to an X-linked recessive deficiency of factor VIII.

▶ Patients develop intra-articular hemorrhages spontaneously or after minor trauma. With repeated episodes of hemarthrosis, patients develop synovial inflammation and proliferation and hyperemia, followed by subchondral resorption and cyst formation and destruction of the cartilage with joint space narrowing. Hyperemia causes epiphyseal overgrowth, osteopenia, and early physeal fusion. The result is findings radiographically indistinguishable from those of JIA.

▶ The most commonly involved joints are, in descending order of frequency, the knee, ankle, elbow, shoulder, and hip. Findings are bilateral, especially in longstanding disease. In the knee, there is femoral epiphyseal overgrowth, squaring of the patella, and widening of the intercondylar notch. In the elbow, there is enlargement of the radial head and the distal humerus and widening of the olecranon fossa. In the ankle, talar slant may develop.

▶ MR helps in the demonstration of subacute hemarthrosis, which is bright on T1 and T2 due to intracellular methemoglobin. Chronic hemorrhage shows a low-intensity rim on T1 and T2 due to fibrosis or hemosiderin. Subchondral cysts are shown well on MR.

▶ Patients may also develop hemophilic pseudotumors. In bones, these appear as expansile, uni- or multilocular lytic lesions that mimic tumors. These most commonly occur in the femur, pelvic bones, tibia, and small bones of the hands.

Next steps in management

Acute hemorrhages are treated with clotting factor therapy.

Further reading

1. Llauger J, Palmer J, Rosón N, Bagué S, Camins A, Cremades R. Nonseptic monoarthritis: imaging features with clinical and histopathologic correlation. Radiographics. 2000 Oct;20 Spec No:S263–S278.
2. Doria AS. State-of-the-art imaging techniques for the evaluation of haemophilic arthropathy: present and future. Haemophilia. 2010 Jul;16 Suppl 5:107–114.

History

▶ 13-year-old with pain after falling.

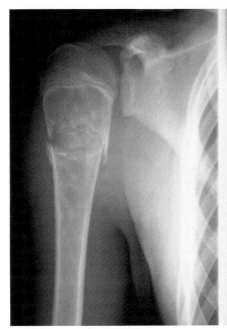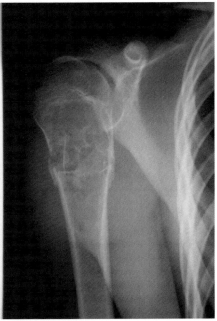

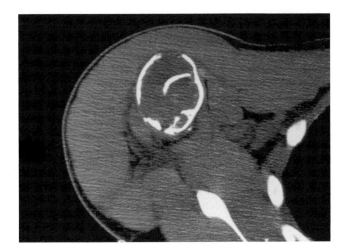

Case 139 Unicameral Bone Cyst (UBC) with Pathologic Fracture

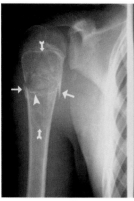 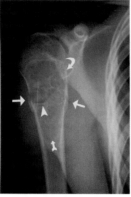 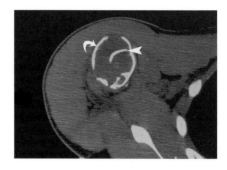

Findings

▸ AP radiographs of the upper humerus (left) show a mildly expansile lytic lesion (tailed arrows) with cortical disruption (arrows). A dense linear fallen fragment of cortex is noted (arrowhead). Endosteal scalloping is seen (curved arrow).

▸ Axial CT image through the lytic lesion demonstrates the fallen fragment (arrowhead) and also shows endosteal scalloping (curved arrow).

Differential diagnosis

The differential diagnosis of a lytic metadiaphyseal bone lesion in this age group without soft-tissue mass or aggressive periosteal reaction also includes nonossifying fibroma, Langerhans cell histiocytosis, unifocal fibrous dysplasia, and subacute osteomyelitis. The finding of a dependent cortical fragment within the lesion indicates the fluid content of the lesion and is pathognomonic for UBC.

Teaching points

▸ In children, solitary or unicameral bone cysts most commonly occur in the proximal humerus, followed by the proximal femur. Most present with pathologic fracture.

▸ UBCs arise in the central medullary cavity of the metaphysis. During the active or growth phase, the cyst increases in size and maintains contact with the physis. In the latent or mature phase, the cyst remains stable in size and the physis grows away from the cyst.

▸ CT and MR are not usually necessary for the diagnosis or management. The MR appearance may be more complex. Typically the cyst contents are similar in signal intensity to fluid, but most patients have a history of pathologic fracture and intralesional hemorrhage, which cause heterogeneity of the signal of the cyst fluid. Fluid–fluid levels may be seen. Generally, only the cyst wall enhances, but thick or small peripheral nodules of enhancement may be noted.

Next steps in management

Casting allows healing of the fracture, but large cysts are treated with curettage and bone grafting or percutaneous injection of steroids.

Further reading

1. Parman LM, Murphey MD. Alphabet soup: cystic lesions of bone. Semin Musculoskelet Radiol. 2000;4(1):89–101.
2. Margau R, Babyn P, Cole W, et al. MR imaging of simple bone cysts in children: not so simple. Pediatr Radiol. 2000 Aug;30(8):551–557.

History

► 6-year-old with bump on head.

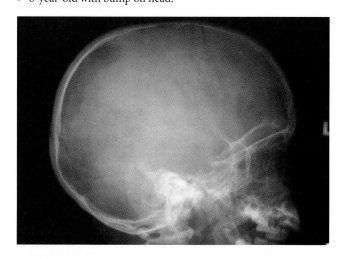

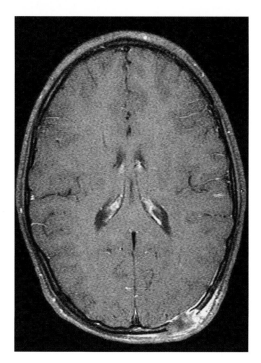

Case 140   Langerhans Cell Histiocytosis (LCH)

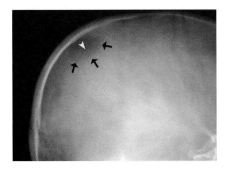 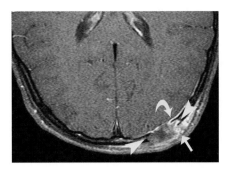

Findings

▶ Lateral radiograph of the skull demonstrates a round radiolucent lesion with differential erosion of the inner (arrowhead) and outer (arrows) tables of the skull (beveled edge).

▶ Axial post-gadolinium T1-weighted MR image shows a soft-tissue mass in the calvarium extending into the scalp (arrow) and causing bone erosion (arrowheads) and dural enhancement (curved arrow).

Differential diagnosis

The particular differential considerations for skull lesions are intra-osseous hemangiomas and dermoid/epidermoid.

Teaching points

▶ LCH is a spectrum of clinical disease due to proliferation of immature dendritic cells originating in the bone marrow. Three clinical patterns of disease are described, although features may overlap. Letterer-Siwe disease is a severe multisystem disease with a fulminant clinical course that occurs in infants. Hand-Schüller-Christian disease is characterized by the triad of radiolucent bone defects, diabetes insipidus, and exophthalmos in young children. Eosinophilic granuloma is an indolent localized disorder of bone or lung in older children and adolescents.

▶ Bone lesions are usually solitary but may be multiple, particularly in children under age 5 years. Any bone may be affected, but the majority of lesions involve flat bones. In the long bones, most lesions arise in the medulla of the diaphysis and cause endosteal scalloping. Lesions can cross the physis.

▶ The radiographic appearance depends on the biologic behavior of lesions. In the fulminating form, the bone lesions may appear as diffuse osteopenia with periostitis. In the acute phase, aggressive symptomatic lesions are lytic with ill-defined, irregular margins. Less aggressive lesions may have continuous smooth periosteal reaction. These lesions may heal spontaneously, becoming more sharply circumscribed and sclerotic. Spine lesions cause anterior wedging or vertebra plana with preservation of the disk space (vs. infection).

Next steps in management

Diagnosis requires biopsy. Treatment ranges from none to chemotherapy for multisystem disease.

Further reading

1. Azouz EM, Saigal G, Rodriguez MM, Podda A. Langerhans' cell histiocytosis: pathology, imaging, and treatment of skeletal involvement. Pediatr Radiol. 2005;35:103–115.

2. Stull MA, Kransdorf MJ, Devaney KO. Langerhans cell histiocytosis of bone. Radiographics. 1992 Jul;12(4):801–823.

History

▶ 15-year-old with chest mass.

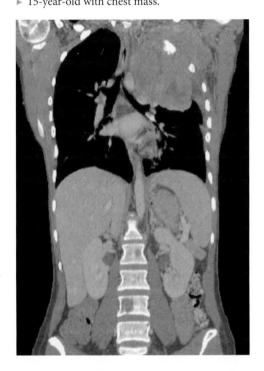

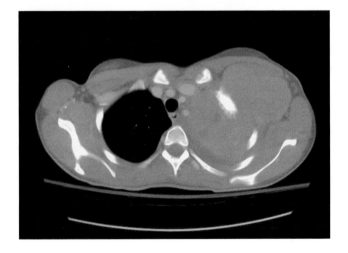

Case 141 Ewing Sarcoma of Rib with Bone Metastases

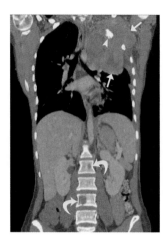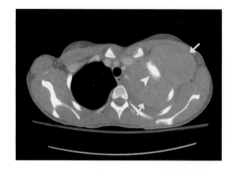

Findings

▶ Coronal contrast-enhanced CT reformation (left) reveals a large mass of the thorax (arrows) surrounding a rib (arrowhead). Also note lytic lesions of vertebral bodies (curved arrows).

▶ Axial CT image shows the mass (arrows) and periosteal reaction of the rib (arrowhead).

Differential diagnosis

A large chest wall mass may mimic a mediastinal mass. The finding of a mass with destruction or periosteal reaction of a rib suggests Ewing sarcoma. Other considerations include Langerhans cell histiocytosis and actinomycosis.

Teaching points

▶ The Ewing sarcoma family tumors (ESFT) include Ewing sarcoma of bone, extraosseous Ewing sarcoma, and primitive neuroectodermal tumor (PNET or Askin tumor). These are primitive small round blue cell tumors that share a common cytogenetic feature—a reciprocal translocation t(11;22)(q24;q12).

▶ The incidence of Ewing sarcoma peaks in children aged 5 to 15 years, and it is more common than osteosarcoma in the first decade. The diaphysis or metadiaphysis of long bones is the most common site, followed by flat bones of the thorax and pelvis.

▶ An ill-defined permeative lytic lesion is the most common radiographic appearance. Cortical bone destruction or aggressive periosteal reaction is typical, often with a multilayered or "onionskin" appearance. There is no calcified matrix and the soft-tissue component is typically underappreciated on plain radiographs.

▶ MR and CT demonstrate a disproportionately large soft-tissue component. MRI yields useful information about marrow involvement. Skip lesions or bone metastases may occur and may be detected with whole-body MR diffusion-weighted imaging, Tc-99m bone scintigraphy, or F-18 FDG PET-CT.

Next steps in management

Tumor staging studies include chest CT, whole-body bone scintigraphy, and bone marrow biopsy.

Further reading

1. Meyer JS, Nadel HR, Marina N, et al. Imaging guidelines for children with Ewing sarcoma and osteosarcoma: a report from the Children's Oncology Group Bone Tumor Committee. Pediatr Blood Cancer. 2008 Aug;51(2):163–170.
2. Mar WA, Taljanovic MS, Bagatell R, et al. Update on imaging and treatment of Ewing sarcoma family tumors: what the radiologist needs to know. J Comput Assist Tomogr. 2008 Jan–Feb;32(1):108–118.

History

▶ 8-year-old girl with pain and swelling after a fall.

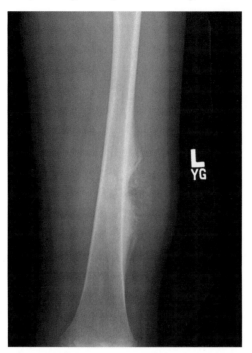

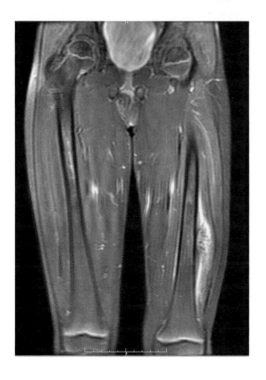

Case 142 Periosteal Osteosarcoma

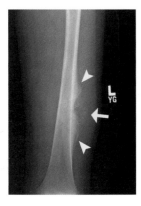 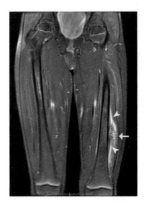

Findings

▶ AP radiograph of the femur (left) shows thickening of the lateral cortex (arrowheads), which is saucerized by a broad-based, soft-tissue mass. Perpendicularly oriented periosteal new bone formation extends into the mass (arrow).

▶ Coronal fat-saturated post-gadolinium T1-weighted image (right) shows the Codman angles (arrowheads), hypointense rays extending into the enhancing mass (arrow), and absence of an intramedullary extension.

Differential diagnosis

The more common diaphyseal tumor in children is Ewing sarcoma, which also causes aggressive periosteal reaction and a soft-tissue mass, but also an intramedullary mass. Langerhans cell histiocytosis also arises in the diaphysis of long bones and may induce aggressive-appearing periosteal reaction, but is primarily an intramedullary mass.

Teaching points

▶ Juxtacortical or surface osteochondromas are divided into three types with distinct imaging appearances and biologic behavior: parosteal, periosteal, and high-grade surface osteosarcoma. Parosteal osteosarcoma is a low-grade malignancy of the metaphysis with excellent prognosis in the absence of deep intramedullary extension. High-grade surface osteosarcoma, an aggressive malignancy arising in the diaphysis, is more likely to invade the medullary canal and carries a much worse prognosis. Periosteal osteosarcoma also arises in the diaphysis but rarely invades the medullary canal and carries an intermediate prognosis.

▶ Periosteal osteosarcoma most frequently occurs in the diaphysis of the tibia or femur. The peak age of incidence is in the second and third decades.

▶ Axial images show the mass surrounds about 50% of the cortex. The well-defined mass demonstrates low attenuation on CT and hyperintense signal on water-sensitive sequences owing to the high water content of cartilage in this tumor with predominantly chondroblastic differentiation. Adjacent reactive marrow changes that are not contiguous with the soft-tissue mass are commonly seen. Actual intramedullary tumor extension is rare.

Next steps in management

Biopsy is necessary for definitive diagnosis.

Further reading

1. Murphey MD, Robbin MR, McRae GA, et al. The many faces of osteosarcoma. Radiographics. 1997 Sep–Oct;17(5): 1205–1231.
2. Murphey MD, Jelinek JS, Temple HT, et al. Imaging of periosteal osteosarcoma: radiologic-pathologic comparison. Radiology. 2004 Oct;233(1):129–138.

History

► 3-year-old girl with left leg pain.

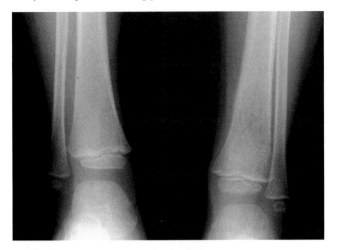

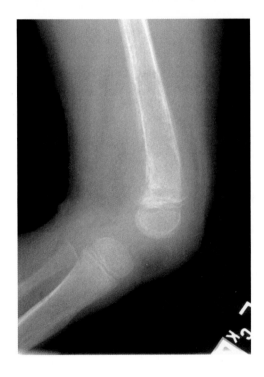

Case 143   Acute Lymphocytic Leukemia (ALL)

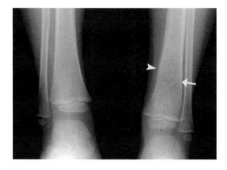 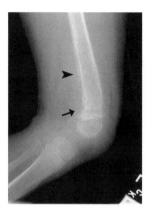

Findings

▶ AP radiograph of the ankles (left) shows a moth-eaten appearance to the left metadiaphysis (arrow) and a layer of periosteal reaction (arrowhead).

▶ Lateral radiograph of the left knee (right) shows ill-defined lucency of the distal femur, periosteal reaction (arrowhead), cortical destruction (arrow), and the suggestion of a soft-tissue mass.

Differential diagnosis

The differential for lytic bone lesions is large but multifocality narrows the differential to leukemia/lymphoma, metastatic disease (usually neuroblastoma), or multifocal osteomyelitis (unusual).

Teaching points

▶ Leukemia is the most common malignancy of childhood, and ALL accounts for 80% of childhood leukemias. Up to one third of patients present with musculoskeletal complaints.

▶ Leukemia in bone produces a variety of radiographic appearances.
- Transverse metaphyseal lucent bands ("leukemic lines")—nonspecific; most common at the knee, distal radius, and proximal humerus
- Periostitis—due to extension of the leukemic cells from the marrow through the Haversian canals
- Diffuse osteopenia or, less commonly, sclerosis
- Focal destructive lesions—chloroma or granulocytic sarcoma in acute myelogenous leukemia; aggressive radiographic appearance
- Permeative or moth-eaten pattern in metaphysis of long bones or flat bones
- Avascular necrosis of femoral head

▶ MR shows diffuse marrow replacement and extension into soft tissue (hemorrhage or chloroma). Replaced marrow appears hypointense on T1 and hyperintense on T2. This finding involving an entire bone suggests leukemia or diffuse metastatic neuroblastoma.

Next steps in management

Additional lesions may be found with plain radiographs or bone scintigraphy. The adrenal glands and retroperitoneum should be evaluated with US for primary neuroblastoma. Diagnosis is made by finding blasts in peripheral blood or bone marrow.

Further reading

1. Miller SL, Hoffer FA. Malignant and benign tumors. Radiol Clin North Am. 2001 Jul;39(4):673–699.
2. Gallagher DJ, Phillips DJ, Heinrich SD. Orthopedic manifestations of acute pediatric leukemia. Orthop Clin North Am. 1996 Jul;27(3):635–644.

History

▶ 3-month-old won't stop crying.

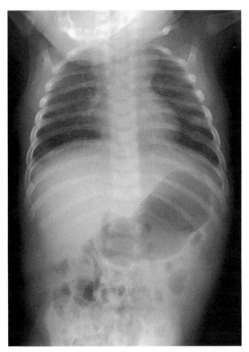

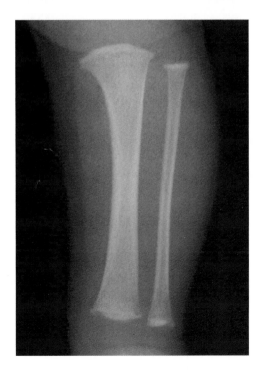

Case 144 Inflicted (Non-Accidental) Trauma

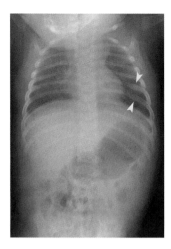 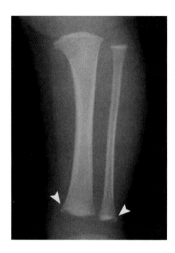

Findings

▶ AP radiograph of the chest (left) shows focal widening of two posterolateral left ribs (arrowheads) representing healing rib fractures.

▶ Radiograph of the left leg reveals oblique linear lucencies in the distal metaphyses of the distal tibia and fibula that extend to the physes (arrowheads), representing classic metaphyseal lesions (corner fractures).

Differential diagnosis

The main differential diagnostic consideration is accidental trauma. Evaluation of the provided history and its consistency with the mechanism of injury and the developmental level of the child, as well as clinical findings, are very helpful in differentiating accidental from inflicted (non-accidental) trauma. Some injuries are commonly related to birth. A clavicular fracture in an infant less than age 1 month is attributed to birth trauma, even if previously unknown. Fractures can occur with mild trauma in patients with osteogenesis imperfecta, but these should be diffusely distributed and not limited to sites of abuse-specific injuries.

Teaching points

▶ Radiographic evaluation of an infant under 18 months of age with suspected inflicted trauma must include a complete skeletal survey (AP and lateral skull; individual AP images of each humerus, forearm, femur, and lower leg; AP chest; AP pelvis; lateral entire spine; and PA hands and feet). Additional views should be obtained of possibly abnormal areas.

▶ Plain radiographs are insensitive for acute rib fractures. Additional oblique images, bone scintigraphy, or repeat radiographs in 1 to 2 weeks can increase detection of rib fractures.

▶ Highly specific skeletal injuries include the classic metaphyseal lesion (corner or bucket-handle fracture) and posterior rib fractures. Bilateral fractures and fractures of different ages are moderately specific for non-accidental trauma.

Next steps in management

A radiologist who encounters an unexpected finding suspicious for child abuse is obligated to contact the referring physician, who will notify child protective services and initiate a complete evaluation.

Further reading

1. Nimkin K, Kleinman PK. Imaging of child abuse. Pediatr Clin North Am. 1997;44:615–635.
2. Offiah A, van Rijn RR, Perez-Rossello JM, Kleinman PK. Skeletal imaging of child abuse (non-accidental injury). Pediatr Radiol. 2009 May;39(5):461–470.

History

► 12-year-old with history of Salter-Harris IV fracture of the proximal tibia.

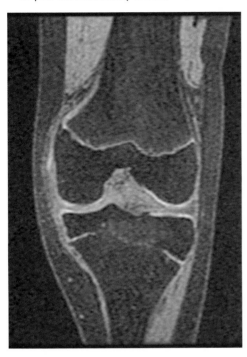

Case 145   Post-Traumatic Physeal Bar or Bridge

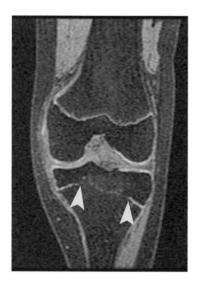

Findings

▶ Coronal fat-suppressed spoiled gradient-recalled echo image of the right proximal tibia shows disruption of the bright line of the physis (arrowheads) with a hypointense bony bridge extending across the physis. Compare to the normal distal femoral physis.

Differential diagnosis

Acute physeal injury shows hyperintense signal on T2-weighted images along with surrounding soft-tissue edema.

Teaching points

▶ Growth arrest or the formation of a physeal bar or bridge complicates about 15% of physeal fractures. The most common site is the distal tibia, followed by the distal femur and proximal tibia.

▶ The risk of growth disturbance complicating physeal injury is dependent upon the type of fracture and on the growth potential of the involved bone. Fractures with more displacement or comminution and fractures that are perpendicular to the plane of the physis are associated with greater risk. Fractures of the distal femur and proximal tibia and fractures in younger patients have greater potential for causing deformity.

▶ Physeal fusion may also complicate avascular necrosis or Blount disease.

▶ Radiographs may initially show physeal narrowing or widening. Bony bridge formation may be seen after a few months. Delayed imaging may reveal leg-length discrepancy or angular deformities due to partial physeal fusion. In advanced cases, the physis adjacent to the bar may appear perpendicular to the normal physis.

▶ MR imaging is more sensitive to early physeal fusion. Three-dimensional fat-saturated spoiled gradient-recalled echo sequences with reconstruction of a map of the physeal plate are useful in guiding surgical therapy.

Next steps in management

Physeal bars that involve less than 50% of the area of the physis can be resected with a good prognosis for resumption of growth. Larger bars may require treatment with corrective osteotomy and/or contralateral epiphysiodesis to prevent further deformity or leg-length discrepancy.

Further reading

1. Lohman M, Kivisaari A, Vehmas T, et al. MRI in the assessment of growth arrest. Pediatr Radiol. 2002 Jan;32(1):41–45.
2. Ecklund K, Jaramillo D. Imaging of growth disturbance in children. Radiol Clin North Am. 2001 Jul;39(4):823–841.

History

▶ 11-year-old with left hip pain.

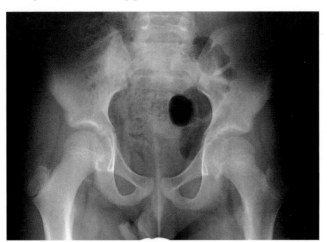

Case 146   Slipped Capital Femoral Epiphysis (SCFE)

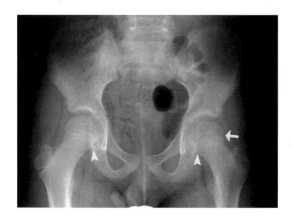
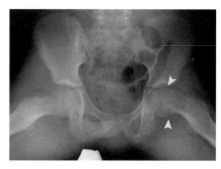

Findings

▶ AP radiograph of the hips (left) shows widening of the left proximal femoral physis (arrow) compared to the right. Additionally, there is loss of the triangular overlap of the medial femoral physis and the ischium on the left compared to the right (arrowheads). These are the signs of SCFE on an AP view.

▶ Frog-leg view (right) better shows the medial slip of the left femoral epiphysis (arrowheads). Normally, the contour of the metaphysis and the epiphysis is congruent as on the right side.

Differential diagnosis

The clinical differential for hip pain includes Legg-Calvé-Perthes disease and septic arthritis.

Teaching points

▶ SCFE is a Salter-Harris I fracture of the proximal femoral physis with posterior slippage of the femoral head epiphysis relative to the metaphysis.

▶ Patients may present with hip or knee pain, which is usually chronic but may be acute. The condition may be bilateral but not usually synchronous. There is an association with obesity and growth spurts. Endocrine conditions predispose patients to SCFE.

▶ Because the displacement is initially in the anterior-posterior plane, findings on AP radiographs in early SCFE are extremely subtle and a high index of suspicion is necessary to prevent a delay in diagnosis. Since it is a physeal fracture, the physis appears widened. The epiphysis maintains continuity with the acetabulum, so that the femoral neck moves away from the acetabulum. Consequently, there is loss of the normal triangular overlap of the medial femoral metaphysis and the ischium.

▶ MR imaging shows joint effusion and edema around the physis, which may predate physeal disruption.

▶ Complications are more likely in cases of delayed diagnosis and include avascular necrosis of the femoral head and early osteoarthritis.

Next steps in management

The goal of treatment is prevention of further slip with in situ pin fixation.

Further reading

1. Busch MT, Morrissy RT. Slipped capital femoral epiphysis. Orthop Clin North Am. 1987 Oct;18(4):637–647.
2. Dwek JR. The hip: MR imaging of uniquely pediatric disorders. Radiol Clin North Am. 2000 Nov;47(6):997–1008.

History

▶ 19-month-old with swelling of both knees.

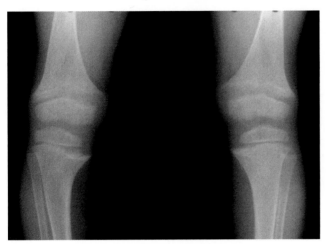

Case 147 Rickets

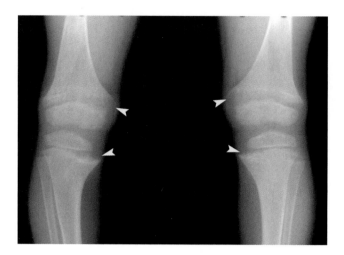

Findings

▸ AP radiograph of both knees shows widening of the zone of provisional calcification and cupping and fraying of the metaphyses of the distal femora and proximal tibiae (arrowheads).

Differential diagnosis

Metaphyseal irregularities in the form of corner fractures or beaks may be seen in inflicted trauma and in Menke kinky hair disease, respectively.

Teaching points

▸ Rickets results from deficient mineralization of osteoid due to deficiency of 1,25-hydroxyvitamin D. Nutritional and vitamin D-resistant (hypophosphatemic) rickets are the most common types, but rickets may be caused by any disease that alters vitamin D absorption or metabolism, including GI, renal, and liver diseases. Nutritional rickets usually presents in infancy but not prior to age 6 months. Risk factors include having dark skin, living in the far north, the practice of covering the skin with clothing or sunscreen, and prolonged breast feeding without supplementation with vitamin D-enriched milk.

▸ The primary abnormality occurs in the zone of provisional calcification where there is decreased mineralization of osteoid, resulting in widening of the zone of provisional calcification. Metaphyseal widening, cupping, and fraying are also apparent. All of the bones become demineralized and the cortical outlines of the epiphyseal ossification centers become indistinct. Left untreated, bowing deformities result.

▸ Radiographic changes are most prominent in sites of the most growth, such as the distal femora, proximal and distal tibia, proximal humerus, and distal radius. Widening of the anterior rib ends may be identified on chest radiographs (rachitic rosary). Skeletal survey for rickets should include AP radiographs of the knees, wrists, and ankles.

▸ In children, renal osteodystrophy is a combination of osteomalacia, rickets, and secondary hyperparathyroidism.

Next steps in management

Serum vitamin D, calcium, and phosphorus levels usually provide the diagnosis. Most patients respond to vitamin D supplementation. Follow-up radiographs are helpful to evaluate response to therapy.

Further reading

1. States LJ. Imaging of metabolic bone disease and marrow disorders in children. Radiol Clin North Am. 2001 Jul;39(4):749–772.
2. Cheema JI, Grissom LE, Harcke HT. Radiographic characteristics of lower-extremity bowing in children. Radiographics. 2003 Jul–Aug;23(4):871–880.

History

► 8-year-old boy with hip pain.

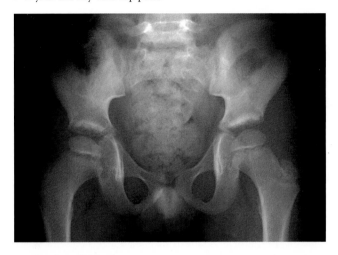

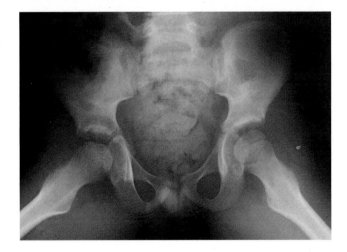

Case 148   Legg-Calvé-Perthes Disease (LCP)

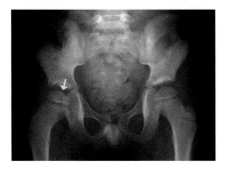 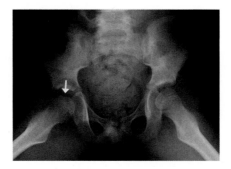

Findings

▶ AP radiograph of the hips (left) shows mild flattening and irregularity of the right femoral head epiphysis (arrow), which is much more apparent on the frog-leg lateral view (right).

Differential diagnosis

Avascular necrosis may be due to systemic diseases, such as sickle cell anemia, or drug therapies, such as steroids. Additionally, fragmented epiphyses may be due to epiphyseal dysplasia. Bilateral findings suggest these other conditions.

Teaching points

▶ LCP is idiopathic avascular necrosis (AVN) of the femoral head that most often affects prepubertal boys (peak 5–6 years of age).
▶ The feared and common sequela is deformity of the femoral head and acetabulum, leading to early osteoarthritis and eventually requiring joint replacement.
▶ LCP is a chronic condition with four stages:
  ▪ Avascular—small sclerotic femoral head ossification center due to lack of blood flow and growth. Articular cartilage is nourished by synovial fluid and hypertrophies. MR and scintigraphy show no flow to the head but marrow edema and increased uptake, respectively, in the neck.
  ▪ Revascularization—subchondral fracture—"crescent sign" followed by collapse, widening, and fragmentation of epiphysis. Widening of the epiphysis leads to coxa magna (wide femoral neck) and deformity of the acetabulum. Disruption of the physis may lead to shortening of the femoral neck. Flow to the epiphysis is seen on gadolinium-enhanced MR.
  ▪ Healing—new bone forms and epiphysis regains height. Lateral extrusion of the epiphysis due to flattening and to cartilage hypertrophy prevents coverage by acetabulum and remodeling leads to a wide flat femoral head.
  ▪ Residual deformity—non-spherical femoral head and altered mechanics leads to early osteoarthritis

Next steps in management

Serial follow-up is performed with plain radiographs. MR also shows the changes to the femoral head, cartilage hypertrophy, disruption of physis, and presence or absence of flow to epiphysis. MR is helpful for early diagnosis.

Further reading

1. Dillman JR, Hernandez RJ. MRI of Legg-Calve-Perthes disease. AJR Am J Roentgenol. 2009 Nov;193(5):1394–1407.
2. Dwek JR. The hip: MR imaging of uniquely pediatric disorders. Radiol Clin North Am. 2000 Nov;47(6):997–1008.

History

► 2-year-old boy with genu varum.

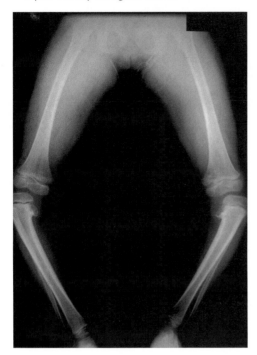

Case 149   Blount Disease

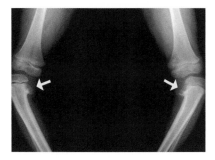 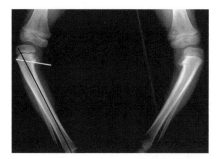

Findings

▸ AP radiograph of the lower extremities demonstrates genu varum (bowed legs). A depressed beak is seen at the medial metaphysis (arrows). The mephaphyseal–diaphyseal angle, the angle between a line perpendicular to a line drawn along the long axis of the tibia (black line) and a line drawn from the medial to the lateral corners of the metaphysis (white line), is more than 11 degrees.

Differential diagnosis

The main differential diagnosis is physiologic bowing that is due to in utero molding and resolves by age 2 years.

Teaching points

▸ Blount disease, also known as osteochondrosis deformans tibiae, is growth suppression of the proximal posteromedial tibia that causes progressive bowing deformity of the knees. The underlying cause is thought to be excessive weight-bearing stress.
▸ There are two types:
  ▪ Early-onset (infantile, 1–3 years)—often bilateral; risk factors include African-American descent, obesity, and early walking
  ▪ Late-onset (adolescent 8–14 years)—usually unilateral; more common in obese boys
▸ Characteristic radiographic appearance of physiologic bowing—symmetric enlargement and mild depression of proximal medial metaphyses (metaphyseal beaking) without fragmentation and thickening of medial tibial cortex. Physiologic bowing does not require treatment but should be followed to ensure it does not become Blount disease.
▸ Characteristic findings of Blount disease, in addition to findings above:
  ▪ Depression, irregularity, or fragmentation of the proximal medial tibial metaphysis
  ▪ Flattening of the medial proximal tibial epiphysis and possibly medial distal femoral epiphysis
  ▪ Widening of medial or lateral physis (early) or vertically oriented medial tibial physis (late)
  ▪ MR shows abnormal signal in physis and adjacent metaphysis. Hypertrophy of the medial meniscus is common. May demonstrate physeal bar.

Next steps in management

Standing radiographs of the entire lower extremities are best for follow-up. MR may be useful to evaluate the physis prior to planned surgery.

Further reading

1. Cheema JI, Grissom LE, Harcke HT. Radiographic characteristics of lower-extremity bowing in children. Radiographics. 2003 Jul–Aug;23(4):871–880.
2. Craig JG, van Holsbeeck M, Zaltz I. The utility of MR in assessing Blount disease. Skeletal Radiol. 2002 Apr;31(4):208–213.

History

▶ 4-week-old with hip click.

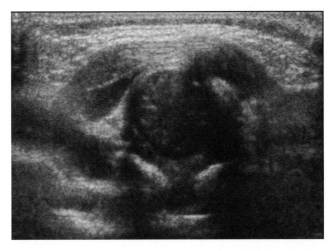

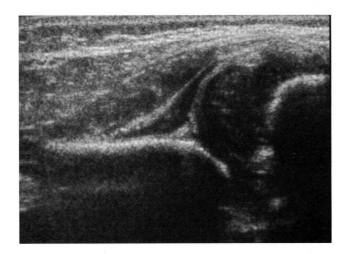

Case 150   Developmental Dysplasia of the Hip (DDH)

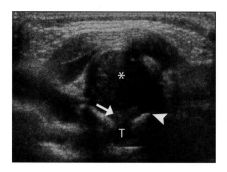 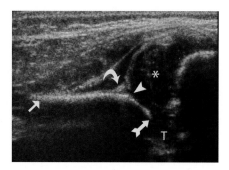

Findings

► Transverse ultrasound image of the left hip (left) shows abnormal lateral displacement of the femoral head (*) relative to the bony acetabulum (arrowhead = posterior ischium) with increased echogenic tissue between the femoral head and the acetabulum (arrow). (T = triradiate cartilage)

► Coronal ultrasound image (right) shows the landmarks of the coronal view of the mid-acetabulum—the horizontal bony ilium (arrow), the echogenic tip of the labrum (curved arrow), and the junction of the bony roof of the acetabulum and the triradiate cartilage (tailed arrow). There is subluxation of the hip with superolateral displacement of the femoral head (*). The superiolateral acetabular margin is slightly rounded (arrowhead) and the acetabulum is shallow (alpha angle < 60 degrees). (T = triradiate cartilage)

Differential diagnosis

Differentiating pathologic DDH from physiologic laxity in very young infants may be difficult. Ultrasound is usually delayed until at least 3 weeks of age.

Teaching points

► DDH is a dynamic spectrum of hip abnormalities with two components—instability and acetabular dysplasia. Instability ranges from subluxable to irreducible dislocation. Risk factors include family history, breech presentation, and oligohydramnios.

► Instability is best evaluated with the dynamic method of Harcke in which the hip is viewed in coronal and axial planes at rest and with the stress maneuver (Barlow). In the axial view, the hypoechoic femoral head normally looks like a golf ball on a tee. With subluxation, the femoral head moves laterally (toward the laterally positioned transducer). In dislocation, the femoral head jumps over the posterior ischium.

► Acetabular dysplasia is best evaluated on the static coronal image of Graf. The femoral head looks like a meatball in a spoon. Normally, the femoral head is more than 50% covered by bony acetabulum.

Next steps in management

DDH is initially treated with a Pavlik harness and followed with ultrasound monthly.

Further reading

1. Harcke HT, Grissom LE. Pediatric hip sonography. Diagnosis and differential diagnosis. Radiol Clin North Am. 1999 Jul;37(4):787–796.
2. Bellah R. Ultrasound in pediatric musculoskeletal disease: techniques and applications. Radiol Clin North Am. 2001 Jul;39(4):597–618, ix.

List of Cases

Index